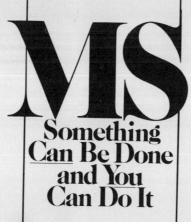

MS
Something Can Be Done and You Can Do It

MS

Something Can Be Done and You Can Do It

A New Approach to Understanding and Managing Multiple Sclerosis

Robert W. Soll, M.D., Ph.D.
Penelope B. Grenoble, Ph.D.

Contemporary Books, Inc.
Chicago

Library of Congress Cataloging in Publication Data

Soll, Robert W.
    MS—something can be done and you can do it.

    Bibliography: p.
    Includes index.
    1. Multiple sclerosis—Nutritional aspects.   2. Multiple sclerosis—Diet therapy.   3. Food allergy—Complications and sequelae.   I. Grenoble, Penelope B.
II. Title.
RC377.S65   1984   616.8'340654   84-1889
ISBN 0-8092-5469-7

Published by Contemporary Books, Inc.
180 North Michigan Avenue, Chicago, Illinois 60601
Manufactured in the United States of America
Library of Congress Catalog Card Number: 84-1889
International Standard Book Number: 0-8092-5469-7

Published simultaneously in Canada by Beaverbooks, Ltd.
195 Allstate Parkway, Valleywood Business Park
Markham, Ontario L3R 4T8 Canada

To my mother and father,
who gave me my start and
encouraged me along the way
RWS

To Professor Jay Gould,
who helped in the beginning
PBG

CONTENTS

FOREWORD

I first met Dr. Robert Soll in 1964. He was my lab instructor in sophomore microbiology at the University of Minnesota School of Medicine. He had finished his neurology residency and was working on the teaching credits which the Ph.D. program in immunology required. He shared with us some of his research on allergic encephalomyelitis and the fluffy white rabbits whose pink ears became pale with cold when the animals were injected with endotoxin. It was obvious then that he had more than a passing interest in multiple sclerosis, "the crippler of young adults."

My own MS had not yet been diagnosed. The strange episodes of tingling and tightness had not yet been given a name. As a matter of fact, I had been told definitely that it wasn't MS because the colloidal gold curve test on my spinal fluid had turned out normal. The symptoms returned, however, and couldn't be ignored. I was referred to a neurologist in private practice who reversed the previous certainty and admitted that I might, indeed, be afflicted with multiple sclerosis. I hurried back to the medical school and sought out Dr. Soll. He listened to my story, considered the facts, comforted me in the way only a truly compassionate physician is able, and advised me of what I could expect and what I might do. "I'm not sure it's MS either, but that's certainly a possibility. Don't listen to the doomsayers," he told me. "When you're down, find me and we'll talk."

I have taken his advice over the ensuing years. Very quickly, he became a mentor and a friend. In my student days, he not only listened to my classroom concerns, but also attempted to expand my understanding of my disease. He explained his theories about endotoxin, basic myelin protein, and the immune response, concepts that were still very new to me at my stage of medical school education. He shared with me the story of Mary Sue that he shares with you in the introduction to this book. Most of all, he confided to me his intent to take on the challenge of MS—and win.

I continued a year after that meeting with Dr. Soll without substantial problems. Then suddenly, during the medical rotation of my junior year, I became ill with strep throat and bronchitis. The vision in my right eye blurred. Again, I sought out Dr. Soll. He considered my symptoms, put me in the hospital, and started treating the infection. Within a few days, I was almost blind in that eye. Retrobulbar neuritis— just one of the many ways MS can manifest itself. The diagnosis was finally made. I was beginning to feel that I didn't have MS—it had me.

Again, Dr. Soll found time for talk and comfort. It is an unfortunate occupational hazard of neurologists that they are frequently called upon to deliver diagnoses of rather dreadful disorders—there are few inconsequential things that can go wrong in the brain and spinal cord. Dr. Soll seemed to deviate from the norm in that he was also very sensitive to the emotional effects of a disease like MS. This attitude made an important contribution to my attitude toward and management of the disease.

When my fever came down, ACTH was started and my eye began to slowly improve. While I was in the hospital, my classmates visited, already convinced that this attack had signalled my withdrawal from medical school. "Tough break," they said; "It's been nice knowing you." Dr. Soll would stop by every morning to start my intravenous ACTH if it wasn't already running. He'd perch on my window sill in the slowly brightening Minnesota dawn and listen for a while—Had I slept well? he would want to know. How was my cough? My eye? Yes, it was OK to be frightened. And then the reassuring, "Don't worry, you'll be back in class by

Wednesday." In the late afternon, he'd come back and perch again. He would take note of my day and then talk about his own day, sharing his thoughts and theories and giving me progress reports on his experiments.

True to his prediction, I was back in class on Wednesday, dressed in my white coat and with my pajama legs rolled up under my skirt. With my triple therapy—antibiotics, ACTH, and Dr. Soll—I graduated from medical school the following year and proceeded to General Rose Memorial Hospital in Denver for my internship.

It was in Denver that I realized how different my experience with MS was from that of other patients. At that time MS was a "wait-and-see" disease. Sometimes the only treatment was a check-up every six weeks. It was not considered an emergency room condition—there was no rush to treat you when your vision began to blur. Not threatened with a life or death situation, your MS could wait until morning. By then, your vision might be gone completely. Various treatment regimens for MS had been in and out of favor: the low-fat diet, ACTH, Vitamin B_{12}, prednisone. There was no generally accepted treatment for MS as there was for strep throat or tuberculosis. MS patients may or may not have been treated with prednisone or ACTH. They may or may not have gotten physical or occupational therapy. If they happened to have a stuffy nose they may have gotten a decongestant, but rarely an antibiotic. I thought I had learned specifics in Minneapolis: "(1) find and treat the infection quickly; (2) treat the MS with ACTH." It was so different in Denver.

Despite my efforts during my internship, my MS symptoms continued. The most dramatic were the sudden episodes of tightening at the waist associated with wobbley legs and a transient episode of "useless hand" syndrome. I also still had occasional trouble with blurred vision. As frightening and depressing as the physical symptoms were, there was also the emotional isolation. My parents, and probably most of my friends, thought I would eventually become an invalid—it was only a matter of time. I made it through my internship and then my residency. When I started working and earning money, I invested some of it against the day when I might become incapacitated. I was determined not to burden my family with the expense of my care.

I had wanted to study gynecology and obstetrics, but, in consideration of my disease, I was convinced to do my residency in pathology (a "nine-to-five" job) and become a board certified pathologist. Later, I was offered a fellowship at Denver General Hospital that enabled me to study my originally chosen specialty. My work now is primarily in prenatal obstetrics, office gynecology, and family planning.

Dr. Soll and I kept in touch over the years. He continued to work with MS, and we exchanged news and information on his research results. We debated theories, swapped success stories, and discussed his move to Waterloo, Iowa, to open the MS clinic. By then it had been 13 years since we had first met.

Then in 1979, sadly but with great confidence, I referred my younger brother to Dr. Soll at his Iowa clinic. Jim had been diagnosed with MS. I went to see him in Waterloo and there experienced firsthand the work with food allergies. Jim concentrated on detecting his allergic foods, and although he found there was little left he could eat, he stuck to his diet and improved. His was the type of MS with frequent exacerbations of walking problems and the ruthless course to a wheelchair, so his improvement was especially dramatic.

Impressed by my brother's progress, I continued to investigate via telephone and letter, and using niacin and water-packed tuna as my initial "diet," I developed a list of "safe" foods that I could eat and could use to sustain myself as I tested the rest of what I ate. (It was a year before I could stand to eat tuna again.) Slowly I developed my allergen-free diet, and my symptoms remained quiet. Thus inspired, I scouted Denver for a neurology resident who might study with Dr. Soll. When I couldn't locate anyone, I went to Waterloo myself, to learn all I could about the allergy elimination diet, about niacin responses, and to continue to increase my knowledge of the enigmatic disease of multiple sclerosis. One day while I was there, a young man—also an MS patient—arrived with a copy of the book that helped make food allergy testing easier, Arthur Coca's *The Pulse*

Test: Easy Allergy Detection. Dr. Soll scanned the book and gave it to me to read. We conferred about its implications, and I started to implement Coca's technique for detecting allergic foods. I stayed in Iowa for almost five weeks, accompanying Dr. Soll on his rounds and assisting him in teaching patients about pulse testing. This and other techniques were incorporated into the food allergy testing process. It was during that time that he confided to me his apprehension that, as a scientist, he was not doing enough to verify his treatment technique. He knew he should initiate controlled studies to clarify his work, "but," he told me, "people come to me for help, and knowing that I can help them, how can I deny any of them my best efforts? How could I relegate any one of them to a control group?"

Dr. Soll left Waterloo later that year to write this book—in the hope of sharing with the medical profession and the MS patient population, the science behind his understanding of the disease and the therapeutic expertise that he had seen could help. He was concerned particularly about people who didn't understand what he was doing and found it too easy to dismiss his results.

I have had my MS for 21 years now. The early times of anxiety are over—finishing medical school, surviving the rigors of an internship, and the challenge of convincing my superiors that, although I did have MS, I wasn't going to die or fall apart. These concerns have been replaced with the confidence that I can keep myself healthy and productive with my now revised triple therapy—diet, antibiotics, and very occasionally ACTH or prednisone in an emergency.

The diagnosis of MS has become easier over the last 21 years. More accurate tests—oligoclonal banding and the VER (Visual Evoked Response) have replaced the colloidal gold curve. It is no longer necessary to make the diagnosis of MS only on the basis of "lesions scattered in time and space"—involvement of different brain and spinal cord locations, episodes separated by months or years that made the waiting for the answer to "What's happening to me?" seem so interminable.

I feel very strongly that the course of my disease would

have been different if I had not been either in Dr. Soll's direct care or influenced by his theories on endotoxin and food sensitivity. During my med school days, we tried to prevent infection or to identify and treat it quickly. We treated runny noses of viral origin prophylactically with antibiotics to prevent their becoming secondarily infected with endotoxin-producing bacteria. We treated new symptoms quickly with ACTH to prevent the progression of blurriness to blindness or numbness of the toes to numbness of the whole leg.

With the recognition of food sensitivity as an endotoxin source, prevention of those exacerbations not associated with obvious infection became a reality.

In December of 1982, I had been without an exacerbation for over three years when I unwisely started eating all the holiday goodies. My vision was blurred again for a while. I hope that's the last reminder I'll need that the diet works.

Back when I was in medical school, women with MS were encouraged not to bear children, but, if they *must* have a family, to adopt. I took that advice, vowing that someday I would "adopt my children housebroken." No longer insecure about the future of my health, I've fulfilled that vow, and for almost four years now I've been the adoptive mother of two lovely blonde daughters, now 10 and 11 years old. Not infrequently one or the other, with visible empathy, will ask, "Mom, don't you feel sad sometimes that you can't eat pickles [or peanut butter or hot fudge sundaes] anymore?"

"Yes, Sweetheart," I answer, nodding, "sometimes I'm a little sad about it, but I'm not sad that I'm feeling good, and I'm really happy that I have you."

I am heartened that this book makes it possible for many others to have the opportunity, as I did, of benefiting from the intelligence, curiosity, dedication, and compassion of my colleague, friend, and physician, Robert Soll.

Marjorie A. Mack, M.D.
Staff Physician: OB-GYN Clinics,
Neighborhood Health Program, City and County of Denver
Private Practice: Office Gynecology and Family Planning,
Mayfair Women's Center, Aurora, Colorado

PREFACE

There are many reasons to write a book. Whichever an author may choose, he or she must believe in the task, because it is no easy doing. We wrote this book because we felt we had assembled a body of information that people might take advantage of.

The practice of medicine has made great strides in this century. It has identified new diseases and has developed drugs and surgeries to treat illnesses that were once fatal. Additionally, we have at our disposal the most sophisticated diagnostic equipment the world has ever known. Because of these advances, we have discovered many answers. Perhaps even more challenging, we have identified as many more perplexing questions.

There are those who believe that some of what medicine has accomplished in the last fifty years has not been all for the good. Their concern is for the alienation of the patient. Have we depersonalized the relationship between the physician and those who seek his care?

We believe that this is too simplistic a view. Medicine has always required a partnership between patient and physician. Perhaps it is true that currently this critical balance has become a bit lopsided. Because of the arsenal of weapons the physician now has at his disposal, it may seem that he is the person with all the answers. From all that ails us, from all of our indulgences, it seems that he can rescue us.

Thus, if there is a difficulty in the advancements of medicine in this century, it may be the divorcing of the individual from his own health concerns. Have we forgotten that our body belongs to us? That it is at least partially our responsibility to keep it healthy? Certainly the physician can patch us up if we become ill and can prescribe therapies to keep us healthy. The rest is up to us. If there is an alternative medicine, as some have claimed recently, it is simple. It is ourselves.

In a specific sense this book is about multiple sclerosis. In another, it concerns you as a person who becomes ill and how you may participate in your recovery. We have approached this challenge from two different, though compatible, perspectives. The first is that of a physician, instilled with the sense of healing. The second is that of a health communicator trained to interpret the advances of science to a complex world.

As with any effort of this scope, many people have contributed. First, the staff of the Soll Neurology Clinic in Waterloo, Iowa, along with the health professionals who treated MS patients at the hospitals in Waterloo. Also, the many patients who accepted the challenge to work at their treatment and to control their MS. Their experiences provide the basis for this book. We also owe thanks to our editor, Mary Eley, herself an MS victim, who guided the book to its conclusion, and to our publisher, Contemporary Books, for their leadership in helping people lead better lives, and to Dr. Jan Robbins, Professor and Head, Department of English Language and Literature at the University of Northern Iowa, for introducing us.

Without the support and enthusiasm of our families, this would have been hard work indeed. Our thanks to Dr. Grenoble's husband, Phillip Myers, who read and initially copyedited the manuscript, and to Dr. Soll's wife, Doris, who transcribed tapes and updated records. Both provided encouragement and guidance throughout the project.

Our goal was to provide you with information you can use. We also hoped to offer some explanation of the disease which is MS. We are enthused that we were able to accomplish both.

Robert Soll, M.D., Ph.D.
Alexandria, Virginia

Penelope B. Grenoble, Ph.D.
Los Angeles, California

AUTHORS' NOTE

The case histories contained in this book are composites of interviews conducted with a variety of individuals. They do not represent the exact lives or experiences of any particular persons.

The information presented here is not meant to replace the advice and counsel of your physician but to complement it. If you are currently under the care of a physician, you should discuss with him any substantial change in your activities or your diet.

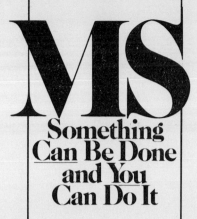

MS
Something Can Be Done and You Can Do It

INTRODUCTION

Sometime in late summer of 1956 Mary Sue Evans, a petite, blond teenager, was admitted to the psychiatric service at a major eastern hospital. The young woman was eighteen years old, and the summer was to have been her transition from high school to college. She had agreed with her parents that she would take the time off, both to give herself a small vacation and to get ready for her first year away from home.

June and July had been routine. Mary Sue and her mother had shopped for new belongings and for some small articles of furniture for her dorm room. They packed up boxes of souvenirs and gave away old clothes. It was a peaceful and yet an exciting time.

August turned out to be a hot, muggy month, and Mary Sue suddenly found that she was not feeling well. At first both she and her parents thought it might be the heat or the excitement of going away to school, except that she seemed to worsen rapidly. Her symptoms included dizziness, disorientation, and extremely irrational and erratic behavior. She would shout at her parents one minute and become overly apologetic the next. She would eat breakfast with her mother to plan their day, only to turn around and announce that she was going back to bed. And throughout this ordeal, she had no idea that she was acting in anything but a rational manner. Mary Sue was one of those young women who had never been sick in her life, nor had she a history of psychological difficulties or emotional problems. Alarmed, her parents first consulted their family doctor. He was unable to establish an explanation for her strange behavior and decided to refer her to a specialist at the local teaching hospital.

After a series of extensive tests, during which Mary Sue's behavior disintegrated even further, the decision was made to admit her to the psychiatric service. More testing ensued, and finally a diagnosis was established. Mary Sue was schizophrenic.

Needless to say, her parents were appalled. The doctor recommended electroshock therapy, which at that time was a standard treatment for schizophrenia. Sadly, after only the first course of shock therapy, Mary Sue went into convulsions. She eventually lost consciousness and slipped into a coma. After days of languishing unconscious in the ward, she was finally transferred to the neurology service. There, after more tests and consultations, it was discovered that this unfortunate young woman was suffering from encephalo-myelitis—inflammation of the brain and spinal cord—which, like other diseases of the central nervous system, is a condition believed to be caused by viral infection. There was, and still is, little medicine can do for this disease, and under the despairing eyes of her family, Mary Sue died a few months later, without ever having regained consciousness.

At the time I, Robert Soll, was serving as an intern in the neurology service. I watched this story slowly unfold in front of me. I particularly remember thinking how frustrating and sad it was that this young woman's doctors had been unable to recognize an organic disease, however untreatable, and had jumped initially to the conclusion that her illness was psychological. I had already become fascinated by the nervous system, and this incident sealed my choice for my medical career: I would specialize in neurology. I concluded from this incident that if seasoned physicians could misdiagnose a known neurological disease as a psychological condition, there must be a lot we don't know and need to understand about the human brain and nervous system.

I went on to finish my medical degree with a specialty in neurology. By that time I had become familiar with the disease that would eventually become my lifelong challenge—multiple sclerosis. I had moved to the Midwest and decided that the basic science I had taken as a medical student was insufficient for the type of work I wanted to do. I had chosen the University of Minnesota because of its reputation in the field of neurology. It was at Minnesota that I first encountered the laboratory experiments that produced the MS model—Experimental Allergic Encephalomyelitis (EAE)—and discovered a number of researchers experimenting with new methods of treating MS patients. Although our work was not a total success, my studies amplified my medical education and my previous clinical experience. I was convinced that a combination of the two approaches—basic science and clinical medicine—would deliver the provocative clues to understanding MS. Science would provide the basis for developing more adequate treatment procedures, and, in return, a patient's response to treatment might return input about the validity of our theoretical assumptions.

Having finished my residency training, I undertook graduate work in immunology and obtained a Ph.D. in that field at the University of Minnesota. After nine years of clinical work at the university I moved from Minnesota to the relatively milder climate of northern Iowa, where I established a neurology practice. I became affiliated with three hospitals in Waterloo and eventually built a small clinic building where patients were received and initially screened.

At the university I worked with a substance called antilymphoblastic globulin (ALG). This is an equine antiserum (a blood serum containing agents of immunity) that has the ability to kill white blood cells and is helpful in suppressing rejection reactions in kidney transplant patients. For this reason, it was thought that it might be useful in suppressing the allergic inflammation of the nervous system, especially in MS patients.

Many of the patients to whom we administered this treatment experienced improvement of their MS symptoms, and we were hopeful that it might be a cure for the disease. You can imagine how disappointed we were when some of the patients, although initially improved, returned a few months later with a severe relapse, apparently triggered by an acute infection. At that time I was also evaluating the relationship between multiple sclerosis and the release of bacterial poisons called endotoxins, which I had first studied at Minnesota. I had long suspected a strong relationship between the presence of an acute bacterial infection and an exacerbation of MS. Because we often were able to dramatically improve worsening MS symptoms merely by treating an ongoing infection, it seemed that elimination of the endotoxin released as a result of such infections could help alleviate symptoms like numbness and paralysis during an MS relapse.

Take, for example, my experience with a young man with multiple sclerosis who was admitted to the Minneapolis VA Hospital. He had developed a high fever associated with the acute onset of paralysis in both legs. Examination proved that he was suffering from bilateral pneumonia. We promptly started intravenous penicillin for his infection and ACTH for the multiple sclerosis, not thinking that the two were in any way related. Within six days he was back on his feet, walking as though nothing had happened. His neurological symptoms cleared more quickly than would have been usual if we had used ACTH alone. This case later reinforced my suspicions about endotoxin's role in the MS disease process. It also convinced me of the importance of advising an MS patient to be under the care of a physician who can regularly check for bacterial infections.

If such infections aren't kept under control, they can initiate a vicious cycle: an exacerbation of MS, for example, that causes a person to lose control of his bladder would also cause him to be unaware of the need to void. This in turn could lead to a clandestine bladder infection of which the person might not even be aware. This infection produces endotoxin, which, as we have seen, may contribute to an exacerbation of MS or, even worse, to the kind of slow deterioration that puts a patient in a wheelchair. If such a cycle is allowed to continue, the individual will eventually reach a point where it would become impossible to control his MS.

As I continued to expand my thinking about endotoxin, I recalled the fact that individuals with multiple sclerosis frequently display a profile of numerous allergies. It would be logical to consider that someone with a sensitivity to airborne allergies might also be hypersensitive to foods. I reasoned that this condition might then cause the absorption of endotoxin from the intestines and an attack of MS. It would also explain why our ALG experiments didn't work. We were indeed killing white blood cells, but they were the wrong kind. We thought we were killing the white blood cells sensitized to myelin while in reality we may have been eliminating the cells sensitized to the person's food allergies, and this later may have enabled them to eat the foods that bothered them without experiencing a reaction. In effect we probably were giving our patients a little holiday from their food allergy problems.

As I was investigating these various factors, I happened to read a newspaper article about an individual who had "cured" his MS. I was drawn to the story by a photograph of a young man, apparently in his early twenties, who was jogging through a field with his wife. The article explained how the young man's wife, dismayed by the incapacitation of his disease, had noticed that he reacted adversely to a wide range of common foods and that she had decided to monitor his food intake. He experienced nausea when he ate meat, egg, and cream, but this disappeared when the foods were eliminated from his diet. Cane sugar also caused him to run a low-grade fever. By correlating his symptoms with his food, she was eventually able to eliminate all the troublesome foods, and he very gradually improved.

Initially, I dismissed the article, chalking it up to a wrong diagnosis. Then I thought about the fever response of rabbits to endotoxin. A rabbit's ears turn cold because its superficial blood vessels constrict with fever. I also remembered that tuberculosis workers, highly sensitized to tuberculin, developed fevers after breathing air accidentally contaminated with powdered TB organisms. Fever, therefore, must be a reaction to a delayed allergy. So, I reasoned further if that young man displayed a fever after eating a specific food, he too must be experiencing a delayed reaction, either to the food itself or possibly to the endotoxin absorbed in his intestines, which had in turn become inflamed from the allergic food reaction.

I also remembered that over the years I had observed that patients with MS often have cold hands and feet, much like the rabbit's cold ears, when they developed an endotoxin-induced fever. My thought was that, since endotoxin was constricting the superficial vessels of the rabbit's ears and thus trapping body heat, something had to be restricting the blood vessels in these patients. It seemed difficult to attribute the coldness to lesions in the nervous system, and most of these patients did not have an infection. My challenge, I decided, was to identify the source of endotoxin.

The intestinal tract may represent a large reservoir of endotoxin, and very small quantities of the substance may be absorbed through a weakened, inflamed intestinal wall as would result from the ingestion of allergic foods. Thus, an infection, which would cause a greater release of endotoxin into the bloodstream, not only causes fever and cold hands and cold feet, but also an acute exacerbation of MS. On the other hand, inflammation of the bowel wall resulting in absorption of endotoxin could produce a slow, cumulative adverse effect day after day, contributing to the slow, downhill course we see so often in MS patients.

I first tested this concept with a middle-aged woman, Mary Fry, who was in the hospital recovering from an acute, ongoing infection associated with an exacerbation of MS. Over the years her legs had been worsening which puzzled me. One day I happened to visit her at lunchtime. I noticed that, along with a full tray of food, Mary had also chosen a large container of yogurt. The yogurt, in fact, was the first thing she ate, and she consumed it with gusto. A light went on in my mind. I had already learned that allergic foods may be addicting. After I left the room, I checked her records. Sure enough, Mary was ordering yogurt with every meal.

I put in an order for a dose of niacin to be given to Mary an hour before each meal. Niacin, or vitamin B_3, has been used for years as a vasodilator in many conditions to improve circulation. It causes a harmless flushing or reddening of the skin because it dilates the blood vessels, usually for about thirty minutes. I had always been puzzled, however, by the fact that while some patients became brilliant red after taking niacin, others showed no reaction at all. Could people be flushing due to a food allergy? I went in to see Mary about midafternoon the next day. She mentioned that she had had an uncomfortable, itchy reaction after both breakfast and lunch and went on to describe the niacin flush. Her reaction suggested that if someone takes niacin before a meal and is allergic to a food eaten at that meal, flushing will occur five minutes to an hour after eating.

Pleased that my hunch seemed to be correct, I explained to her that I was trying to determine whether something she was eating was bothering her. She wasn't enthused. I went back the next day, and she asked me to stop the niacin. I stopped the yogurt instead. I went back the third day, and she scolded me, "Dr. Soll, you didn't stop the niacin." I told her that no, I had stopped her yogurt. "Yes," she said. "I noticed that, but I didn't flush." We discussed it a bit further, and finally she agreed that she might be having a problem with dairy products. She wanted to know whether I thought it was the bacteria or the milk in the yogurt that was affecting her. We decided to test it and tried skimmed milk. Mary flushed. Eventually, she went home with a "prescription" to avoid dairy products, and after that the use of niacin became routine with my MS patients. I found that although virtually all the patients stopped flushing when they stopped eating the foods that seemed to be causing the reaction, those foods varied with each patient. I concluded that the flush had to be resulting from an intolerance the patients had developed to a food, regardless of the fact that they had not experienced an obvious disagreeable reaction to that food. After discovering which foods caused individuals to flush, I eliminated them from their diet and they gradually began to feel better.

If I had any doubts about food allergies, a case several months later dispelled them. In September 1977 a very concerned Tom Gardner brought his critically ill wife, Dorothy, to me. Three years earlier she had quit her job because of her growing paralysis. Toward the end of that year, however, she was able to deliver a healthy baby. Soon after that, the frequency of her MS symptoms was such that her legs were almost completely nonfunctional. By the time I admitted her to the hospital, she was completely paralyzed on her left side, and only minimal movement remained in her right arm and leg. Her speech was hardly understandable— she could barely articulate a few audible sounds. During the first twenty-four hours in the hospital she continued to get worse so rapidly that I was afraid she might stop breathing. The situation was so bad that I warned her husband and her mother that she might die.

Transferring her to the intensive care unit, I immediately started conservative supportive care and treated her for a bladder infection. She also received intravenous ACTH with which I was trying to control her MS. She was fed through a tube into her stomach, but instead of food, we gave her Vivonex, which is essentially a combination of purified amino acids and glucose manufactured by Norwich-Eaton. She thrived on this nutrient, and over the next month she gradually gained strength, despite the fact that I had to discontinue the ACTH after only a few days because her blood sugar rose to diabetic levels. This meant the only treatment left to me was diet. Although it was several weeks before she was able to utter any understandable words, she remained conscious the entire time and never required respiratory assistance.

As Dorothy gained strength, I decided to start her on some type of food. The first food we tried was chicken, which I thought would be rather bland. We ground it up and fed it to her through the tube. She immediately developed severe diarrhea, so I switched to fish, which she was able to tolerate. I later discovered that chicken was a frequent menu item at her home. Over the next several months we expanded her diet to include potatoes, broccoli, and lima beans. By early December, she was able to go back to the regular ward. When she had regained enough of her power of speech, she and I talked about her ordeal. She told me that she didn't know where she was and, in fact, at first thought she was in her bed at home. Apparently, one of the shelves in the hospital room reminded her of furniture in her bedroom. I was surprised at this, and I asked what was the last thing she remembered. She told me she remembered going to her grandmother's funeral, which had taken place eleven months before. In effect she had no memory of that whole year. Dorothy finally left the hospital in January 1978. By that time she could move all her extremities, dress herself, and stand and walk with only the minimal assistance of a walker. Her longest previous remission of MS had lasted only three weeks and always required the administration of ACTH. During the time she was in the hospital—with her only treatment being diet—she had been improving for four months. She went home, gradually added more foods to her diet, and has now gone four years without an exacerbation, except for a brief setback one spring as the result of the flu.

My experience with Dorothy Gardner confirmed my suspicions about the importance of diet to the point that I vigorously monitored the diet of all my patients. Those who came in with severe exacerbations of MS were easy to treat because they were a captive audience. Since they were in the hospital, I could administer Vivonex and explain food allergy to them. It also facilitated administration of niacin to help confirm their food allergies. Once we had their systems cleaned out, it was not difficult to develop a diet and keep them on it—because they couldn't order any food except what was on their charts. Without doubt, the positive experiences they had in the hospital motivated these patients so that when they went home they stayed with their new dietary regimen.

Our entire practice did not, however, focus on acutely ill

patients. Some had their MS at least under temporary control and visited us with the hope of learning how to keep it that way. Although everyone was given the same information about diet and infection, it was more of a challenge to treat these individuals, because their need for care wasn't as acute. They returned home, perhaps wrote to us a few times, and either had the motivation to stay with their diet or gradually fell off. In the early days of this treatment the idea of using a therapeutic diet to control disease had not received the public attention or acceptance that it has recently. Therefore, I gained more experience, especially with the "outpatients," who were not acutely ill and thus not as motivated, I realized that I needed to do two things.

First, I decided it was essential that I organize my thoughts on MS and develop my treatment in a way that others might be able to take advantage of it. A patient who is attempting to manage his disease as I've suggested needs the guidance and aid of his personal physician. If he is using Vivonex to clean out his system, for example, he should be monitored by a doctor. Likewise anyone with MS should be routinely checked for infection. But I knew, however, that if I made either recommendation, I would have to set down my theory and treatment in understandable terms. My second realization was that the time had come to transmit my findings to other members of the scientific and clinical world, as well as to MS patients, in the hope that other people interested in this subject might be able to expand and contribute to my approach. The result of both of these resolutions is this book. In order to complete the manuscript, I recognized the painful necessity of temporarily closing my practice.

My MS case load during my six years of medical practice in Waterloo, Iowa, was 660 patients, out of a total of more than 2,000. I saw perhaps one-third exclusively on a one time basis only; either their MS was not very extreme or the distance between our clinic and their home was too great to allow a sustained relationship. It is difficult to follow closely patients in a specialized practice such as mine because patients came from all parts of the country. Additionally, when I introduced the concept of food allergies in 1978 perhaps 75 of our 440 regular MS patients dropped away. They were concerned that maintaining the type of dietary regimen I was recommending would interfere too much with their quality, or enjoyment, of life. Of the other patients who started on the dietary program, I would estimate that approximately one-half have maintained the allergen- and infection-free lifestyle I recommended as the best opportunity to control their MS. As a result, the majority of them have experienced very few problems with their disease. They have all told me, however, that it has not been a lark. If I were to ask why, they would answer that the dark times are "falling off the wagon." Therefore, I feel extremely fortunate that we have been able to include the motivational chapters in this book. During those early years I was so busy trying to keep my patients well that I didn't have time to become informed of strategies to help them maintain new lifestyles after they left my care. In this regard I'm grateful for the input Dr. Grenoble has provided on this part of the treatment therapy as we've presented it here.

The one aspect of those years that disappoints me is that I was not able to fulfill my original quest of molding science with medicine. Although I was trained as a basic scientist as well as a physician, when it came down to dealing with patients, I was motivated to exert my best efforts to help them achieve maximum health despite their disease. My original goal of classical research succumbed to the physician's mandate to heal the sick. Thus, we don't present a range of verifiable data to prove conclusively that those who adhered to this program did better than those who didn't. Once I saw the effectiveness of the diet and controlling infection, along with physical therapy and interpersonal support, I could not withhold any aspects of this program from any of my patients. The double-blind studies, which would conclusively verify our work, remain to be accomplished, which is, as I said, one of the primary reasons we chose to write this book. My scientific consciousness has finally caught up with me.

I can, however, tell you that, of the original two-hundred-plus patients whom I started on this program, I am in regular contact with fifty. Some have been patients for as long as seven years. These people routinely report to me and ask to be kept up to date on refinements in their treatment. They have stuck by their new lifestyles and have experienced minimal problems with their MS. In the area of lifestyle change a 25-percent compliance rate is not only heartening, it's almost unheard of.

The development and publication of this book completes the cycle activated by the death of Mary Sue Evans almost thirty years ago. Hopefully, my experiences with MS and its relationship to infection and food allergy as contained in these pages will stimulate other researchers and practitioners interested in MS and its related disorders. Certainly, it demonstrates the validity of providing multiple sclerosis patients with alternatives to the conventional approach of asking them to sit back and wait for a cure—or the next exacerbation of their disease.

1

WHAT IT MEANS TO HAVE MULTIPLE SCLEROSIS

A small blue-and-grey airplane drops from under the low-hanging cover and completes a routine landing on the concrete runway. The plane taxis quickly out of the way of a 727 heading for takeoff and comes to a stop in front of a deserted commuter gate.

Someone opens the door from inside. A muffled ground attendant waddles over, puts wooden blocks under the wheels, and then makes a job of pulling down the four-step ramp. The first passenger off the plane is a middle-aged man dressed in a leather coat and wearing a hunting cap. He unbends his way out of the small space, swearing at the gust of frigid air that immediately engulfs him. At the bottom of the four steps he slips on a pair of leather gloves and, his walking stick in hand, heads off for the terminal.

The plane's few passengers quickly fill the tiny baggage area with the noise of their efforts to keep warm. The wait for the baggage stretches from fifteen minutes to twenty, then to twenty-five. Finally the same attendant who opened the plane door appears in the lobby to make an announcement. He tells them that there's been a problem with the luggage "at the other end" and their bags will be along on the next flight, which is due at noon the next day. Groans mix with the foot-stomping and arm-slapping as people try to decide what to do.

The man in the leather coat heads to the lobby phone and calls a cab and then waits for another thirty minutes. Irritated, he makes another call, this time to the clinic.

"Hello, this is Peter Samuels. My luggage is missing, and the taxi isn't here yet, and I'm afraid I'm going to be very late for my appointment. Please tell them I'll be there in about forty-five minutes."

The voice at the other end of the phone confirms his message and indicates that she'll pass it on.

In another few minutes the taxi arrives, picks up its passenger, and starts for downtown Waterloo.

December in Waterloo, Iowa, is not inviting. The trees look naked, waiting for their first protective covering of snow. The streets are glazed with ice, which makes driving, and walking, difficult. Clouds hang low on the horizon and cast a grey shadow over the landscape. The going's not easy in Waterloo at this time of year. Unlike some of the lush health spas in this country and in Europe, Waterloo hardly seems a place you'd visit to regain your health.

Peter Samuels' destination is a large white building across from the hospital. Suzanne Baccone is already there. She's well prepared for the Iowa cold, dressed in blue jeans, a ski sweater, and a down vest. As she moves across the room to greet Peter, she whisks off her wool hat, shaking out her long blonde hair. Peter sheds his hat and coat, and they sit down together on opposite sides of a small metal conference table.

Suzanne speaks first.

"It must have been six years ago that we finally figured out that I had MS. Jack and I hadn't been married very long then. But anyhow, he was a wonderful husband; he had a good job, and we had one of our two adorable children. (I'll take 60 percent of the credit for them as long as Jack isn't here.)

The multiple sclerosis started with a numbness in the bottom of my feet, which pretty quickly spread up my legs.

Then I started to lose control of my bowels and my bladder. I thought I'd better do something about it, so I went to my gynecologist. He said it was nerves. Then I went to my GP, and he said the same thing. The gynecologist took me off my birth control pills, and my GP gave me Valium. Needless to say, neither helped. Actually the symptoms got worse. I became completely numb to my waist. It was awful, really. I didn't even know when I had to go to the bathroom. I just went in and sat down on the toilet and listened for the sound. Then I cleaned myself up and left. Of course I had to check the time because I knew I had to come back in two hours.

"Sure, I was very frightened. You know how it is when something's wrong with you and you don't know what it is or what to do about it. I was driving everybody around me slowly crazy. Nobody *knew what to do, and it seemed to be getting worse so fast. I remember I was sitting in the kitchen one morning just looking out the window, asking myself over and over, 'What am I going to do? What's going to happen to me?' Finally I got up from the table. I don't even remember how I decided to do this, but I picked up the phone and called the information operator. I asked her if she had a listing for a neurologist in Iowa. She said there was one in Waterloo, and she gave me a number. I called, and they answered. I can't even remember being surprised.*

"The next thing I knew I was in the hospital having all those tests, which made me even more frightened. My gynecologist and GP hadn't seemed to take me very seriously. But everyone in the hospital seemed to be very concerned. Finally, after a couple of days and a lot of tests, Dr. Soll came into my room and said very simply, 'I think you have multiple sclerosis.'

"It was horrible at first. I had thought of MS because I have two cousins that have it. But after he told me what was wrong and before I could get too upset, he said, 'I think I can help you.' That's when I started to win the battle of MS."

Peter Samuels sits quietly, listening to her story. He knew something was wrong when he was in medical school. Initially he tried to blame his dizzy spells and loss of balance on an inner ear infection. When his self-diagnosis and treatment didn't work, he gave up and went to the medical staff. By then he couldn't read.

"When you sit and stare at the page for a couple of hours and realize that you've made it through only a few sentences, then you know something's wrong. But when they finally came in with the diagnosis, which obviously I suspected, it was like hitting me over the head with a hammer. I could feel my dreams fading.

"I had made the decision to become a doctor very carefully. I'd been in the service and had bummed around. Now it appeared that my goal was slipping away. Without being able to read, how was I going to get through medical school? I was shattered. I'm an emotional person, and I don't mind telling you that I was furious at the horrible hand I felt life had dealt me. I also have this big thing about being independent. I have a very difficult time asking people for help, regardless of whether or not I need it. I vowed that I was still going to become a doctor, even if I could work only a few days a week.

"They gave me what they could, but I just continued to get worse. My walk was pretty unsteady, and I didn't have much stamina. I was mostly afraid that my hands would go and I wouldn't be able to do delicate X-ray work. I kept going over and over the same thought—I had gone to medical school by choice, because I wanted to help people—but obviously I didn't choose to get MS. I was angry, so I tried to avoid acknowledging that I was sick, which, of course, was impossible. It looked to me like I was being locked in by the disease, which is actually what happened until I decided to do something about it.

"Dr. Soll and I figure that now I'm at about 60 percent of my total capacity. If I'd started this when I was first diagnosed in 1969, I'd probably be at 90 percent now. I still can't read very well, but I am a doctor, and I can see well enough to know there's a light at the end of the tunnel. Most of all, there's no doubt in my mind that if I hadn't started this treatment, I'd be retired by now; maybe not in the real sense, but in all that matters—old and tired in my heart and soul."

Philadelphia is half a continent away from Waterloo, Iowa,

but the problems of MS patients are the same. Janet Myerson is sitting in her comfortable suburban living room. She tells her story as if she's talking about someone else.

"In August this city can be very hot and wet. That particular day, the afternoon sun was beginning to get to me. I was daydreaming about being in the backyard, watching the kids jump in and out of the swimming pool.

"My feet hurt, and my nails needed doing, and Nat was going to be home early—I can't remember why—and we were supposed to go to dinner with some friends. I was talking to myself about collecting money for the MS Society. 'What,' I asked myself, 'am I doing this for anyway? Can't they get people to give real money? Why rely on housewives like me to trudge around shaking these silly cans in our neighbors' faces?' I came to the conclusion that maybe not enough people understand MS. If I'd thought about it, I probably would have had to admit that I didn't either. But I remember thinking that collecting was a kind of pay-back for my own life, which I thought was pretty good.

"That was before I got sick.

"We had been in Florida, Nat and I, on an unusual vacation for just the two of us. I noticed a numbness in my left leg when we were there, but I really didn't pay too much attention to it. It was hot and we were on vacation—you know how you tend to do too much. When we came back I started in on my usual schedule, teaching, driving the kids around, going to my aerobics class. It was in aerobics that it showed up. First I couldn't lift my left leg all the way up. A week or so went by, and then I couldn't move it at all. I wasn't alarmed, but I thought I should see a doctor. We went to a family friend first, but he didn't want to make a diagnosis until they'd completely worked me up. So he admitted me to one of the big local teaching hospitals. Among lots of other tests, they did a Cat Scan and a spinal. I knew it had to be something neurological, and I might even have suspected MS, but everybody was so vague."

Janet's husband comes in carrying some glasses and a bottle of Perrier. He continues the story.

"You have to understand that she was pretty bad by then.

By the time we got her to the hospital, she could hardly walk. They wouldn't tell us anything, and we were both getting a little scared. Every day we would ask the doctors, 'Is it MS?' They'd answer, 'No, no; we don't know what it is, but don't worry.'

"Finally, one day, after she'd been in the hospital a week, one of the doctors came into her room. My mother was sitting with her. They've both been great—my mother and father. Anyhow, this doctor walks in and says to her, 'You have MS; I'm sorry.'"

Janet grins as she thinks about that day.

"I don't really remember how I reacted. My mother-in-law had more presence of mind at that moment and asked him right out, 'Well, what do we do about it?' His answer? 'Take her home and call me in a week.'

"I thought she was going to hit him. 'Of course we'll take her home,' she said. 'But what do we do about it now?' 'Nothing,' he answered. 'There's nothing you can do about it. MS is a funny disease. It can go away in three days, or it may take three weeks or three months. It may never go away. But it won't kill her.' I think that was the worst day of my life—it had all happened so fast. Nat came in to help me get ready to go home, and we cried in each other's arms. It had only been less than a month since I'd first noticed the symptoms. Four weeks ago we'd been swimming and jogging in Florida.

"My doctors implied that if I went home and went to bed, I'd be all right. Well, of course I got worse. At that time my kids were two and four. Before, we had always taken pains to do things as a family, but the MS almost totally cut me off from the kids. My world was the bedroom. They'd come in to see me every day, but I couldn't do anything for them. I couldn't even go to the bathroom by myself. Nat had to lift me out of bed and carry me to the bathroom. He had to dress me and even feed me. We had help in the house all the time. I especially liked the little Irish girl who came and took care of me every day. I remember she used to bring this jar of rose milk and rub me with it.

"Both Nat and I were just lost. All our lives we'd solved our problems by facing and analyzing them and then evaluating

our options. With MS, they told us nothing would work—you know, that we should forget it. But I couldn't understand how you'd do that, forget it. I was very concerned about the kids, but I vowed I wouldn't take care of them from a wheelchair, although I had no idea how we . . . how I was going to do it."

Nat elaborates:

"Those were terrible times. The poor kids were so confused. They watched her sinking. They would come out of her room and ask me, 'Why is Mommy crying?' What could I say? The worst part was that I couldn't stop crying either. Both of us felt like we were sinking down into some horrible hole, continually falling, farther and farther down into this horrible darkness. My God, I hate to think what our life would have been like."

The problems of an MS patient start at diagnosis, which is actually a problem in itself. Multiple sclerosis can perplex a physician as much as it confuses his patient. There are no conclusive tests for the disease; in fact there is only one procedure which has been reasonably reliable—identification of myelin particles in the spinal fluid. This can be considered somewhat radical, however, in that it must be done in the hospital. Some physicians may thus be reluctant to frighten an already distraught patient. Other doctors may not want to expose patients to unnecessary risks.

There is the additional complication that, although well over half a million people in this country suffer with MS and MS-related afflictions, many doctors have not had a great amount of experience with the disease. This partly results from the fact that multiple sclerosis has confounded the medical profession ever since it was first identified. Only now is medical science beginning to discover clues to this and other diseases of the immune system. Additionally, the clinical course of multiple sclerosis is far from predictable. Some people have an initial attack and go steadily downhill—in the presence or absence of any treatment—while others never have another attack. Still more people will face the most common pattern of a lifetime of exacerbations and remissions.

There is no doubt that, at its worst, MS can be a devastating disease. The rapid onset of its symptoms is dramatic in itself. An individual can seem to become incapacitated almost overnight, like Janet Myerson. Others bumble along as Suzanne Baccone did, going in and out of the hospital with a varying pattern of symptoms that makes it impossible to conduct a predictable and normal life and causes considerable emotional turmoil, for both the patients and those around them. The emotional difficulties Peter Samuels experienced in his battle with MS illustrate the psychological as well as physiological effects—fractured lives, sometimes never to be recovered.

Physicians may also shy away from a conclusive diagnosis because of their sense of the enormity of the disease. This well-intentioned attempt to protect the patient from bad news has just the opposite effect on an individual who has been living with curious and often frightening symptoms and is anxious for answers. More often than not, a patient suspects that there is something very wrong long before his physician tells him what it is.

Cindy Morse, a young Air Force wife, found herself continually bothered by a tingling in her left arm. She and her husband had just moved to New Hampshire, and she thought it might be the change in weather. It gradually spread to her leg, however, and soon to her whole left side. She decided to see a doctor. He ran a series of tests, while her symptoms continued to worsen.

Cindy describes her experience with her doctor:

"When he finally told me that my symptoms were the result of multiple sclerosis, I whispered secretly to myself, 'Thank God; at least now you know you're not out of your mind.' I knew it anyway, because my grandfather had it. I watched him die with it.

"I think that's the part that really bothered me. After the doctor explained that he had MS, my grandfather asked him what he could expect. My grandmother said the doctor told him he could expect to live seven years. She said he died seven years later to the day. Actually, I remember seeing him go steadily downhill. First he used a cane, then he had a wheelchair, then he just went to bed.

"When I questioned my doctor about what to expect, he answered, 'There's nothing we can do for you. MS is a very funny disease. Just go home and try to live a normal life.' All these thoughts started going through my head. I kept thinking about my grandfather. And I imagined myself doing just what he did. By the time I had finished my scenario, I had myself from a wheelchair to bed, and finally dead—all in less than ten years.

"I asked the doctor when I would get the use of my hand back. He said, 'Well, maybe you will and maybe you won't.' Then he repeated, 'Just go home and be normal; try to lead a normal life.' Normal? How could I do that? He did give me some pills—cortisone—and told me to take them when I thought I needed them.

"I guess if I think about it, I don't really blame him. I know my experience isn't unique, that lots of other people go through the same thing. I played his game for awhile; I took my pills and diligently watched for signs of decline. One problem was that every time I stopped taking the pills, the MS came back just as bad as ever. So, slowly but very determinedly, I continued to live out my grandfather's legacy.

"Finally, one day—I don't know why—I said to myself, 'You know, you just don't believe this. If you can dream up this negative stuff, then you can darn well get some positive thoughts together.' Actually I decided there had to be something I could do. And it turned out there was. I had spun around in circles for almost a year. Boy, am I glad I finally got off that merry-go-round."

And so we have another reason why a physician may find it difficult to deliver a conclusive diagnosis of MS. After he's told the patient what the problem is, he then has to tell him there's nothing he can do for him. Obviously this can be debilitating for both the physician and the patient. There is the additional complication that multiple sclerosis can produce symptoms similar to those of other diseases and disorders. The physician will want to be sure that he is not misdiagnosing a brain tumor or a stroke, a condition like intoxication from heavy metals, a metabolic disease such as diabetes, or even a degenerative disease in a chronic, progressive form. This is particularly important because there are established and effective treatments for many of these.

A final problem complicating the MS diagnosis is that its pattern of exacerbations and remissions can make it difficult to determine that a patient does have MS. Obviously this can be frustrating if a person visits the physician, describes symptoms he has recently experienced, but appears to be symptom-free at the time of the visit. In the absence of symptoms, and with few diagnostic tools at his disposal, the physician could be left to conclude that the patient isn't ill, at least at the time he sees him. His patient, however, knows differently. The usual outcome of this difficulty is that the patient, frightened by the severity of his symptoms, continues searching for a diagnosis, which he may or may not find.

The confusion resulting from this quest for a diagnosis is amplified when the patient asks, "What's next?" Frequently, in a well-intentioned attempt to be realistic, the doctor describes a disease with a slow but inevitable decline into a bedridden existence. The prospect of being condemned to a life that will slowly but surely be shut down is made even worse if the patient is told there is no cure for the disease and no effective treatment for its incapacitating symptoms. The medical profession has long considered hope essential to the healing process. But what could be more defeating and less motivating than to say to a patient, "You have a horrible disease that we don't know much about; its symptoms aren't predictable; we have no medicine we can give you, and there's not much we can tell you to do for yourself"? Even the most confirmed optimist would be challenged.

Suzanne Baccone describes how she felt before she was finally diagnosed:

"I was in an absolute panic because of not knowing what was wrong with me. When I called the information number and asked for a neurologist, I didn't even know if we had one in Waterloo. I was absolutely terrified that it was going to get worse, whatever it was, before I could get to a doctor who could tell me what to do about it. Looking back on it now, even though it still isn't funny, I must have been a terrible

nuisance to my family, running around in a daze like I was. Of course, they were as scared as I was.

"I still get that reaction now, when I slip up and the MS comes back. It's like, whammo, and my vision gets blurry. I've had three really bad attacks since we started on this. Three times I was in the hospital. One time I called Jack and said, 'I think I am going to die. What can we do?' And, of course, we couldn't do anything then. I had fallen off my regimen. Dr. Soll had to do everything so he could get me back where I could start again. He got the exacerbations under control, and I went home. He kept telling me, 'We've got to take it one step at a time.'

"So, over the years I keep relearning my lesson, and I continue to improve slowly. I definitely haven't gotten any worse. Sometimes I think that maybe I'm nervous—well, not nervous exactly, but high strung—and then that's probably when I put myself in danger. I slip up, and then it hits me. But you know, when I started this treatment, we were looking for a nursing home. I was actually going to give up and go into a nursing home. My kids . . . I get chills when I think of it. What would have happened to my kids? And Jack was ready to get a divorce. I was in such bad shape, and there seemed to be nowhere to look for help.

"My life would have been totally different. I wouldn't have had any life. And someone else would be raising my kids right now. I shudder when I think about that. But then again, not everyone is as lucky as I am—do you suppose?"

2

COPING WITH A MYSTERY DISEASE

"Controlled. That's the word I was thinking of. Controlled by that damn disease."

Peter Samuels is lying on a battered couch in his small, cluttered study. The room is littered with magazines and books, most of which are concerned with Peter's interest in the odd diseases and conditions of mankind. A few lost souls of literature are scattered here and there, along with an occasional biography. A portable tape recorder sits on Peter's desk like an intruder in this inner sanctum of the printed page. The walls are covered with photographs of the Samuels family, a few of the older ones testifying to Peter's successful college football career. The room smells of wood polish and dust. The only other decorations are a deer head hung above the desk and a rack of expensive but long-neglected pipes.

Peter is talking about the effects of multiple sclerosis on his marriage.

"When you buy a piece of merchandise—an appliance or maybe even an automobile—you expect it to function in a certain way. Say it doesn't work; maybe it's even a complete

dud. What's your likely reaction? You want to get it fixed, of course. You might even want to take it back and get a new one. Most of all, you're probably angry. You bought the damn thing in good faith, and now you want it to work.

"That's how it is with MS. Take marriage. Most likely when you got married you had a vision of the rosy fairy tales people told you about—that everyone lives happily ever after, bliss from the word go. Of course after a while everybody finds out that there are problems and challenges. Life, after all, has its ups and downs, and you work these things out—until you come to a really big challenge like MS.

"You try to fix it, like the rest of your problems, but nobody has any answers. It's not like a car or an appliance, which you can have repaired or replaced. You can't do that with a marriage threatened by incapacitation or disease. I guess you can solve the inconveniences that result from MS, but that takes a lot of faith on the part of your partner. There's always the chance that he or she will say, 'Yeah, well, I didn't buy that, you know.' And then where are you? Stuck. A person with MS lives with the fear that the husband or wife will wake up someday and say, 'I didn't marry you with MS, I don't want you like this, and I'm getting out.' I think one of the things that leads to this kind of reaction is the partner's apprehension of not being able to handle the situation. That kind of fear can override the love and commitment that motivated two people to get married in the first place.

"Luckily, that didn't happen to me. Susan has stood by me, even though it wasn't too long after we got married that they diagnosed the MS. I would guess that the most difficult time for us was when she went back to work. I've always been able to work, even in the worst of times, but she thought she'd better get a job anyhow, because we weren't sure how long I'd be OK."

Suzanne Baccone talks about her experience with her husband:

"Your life changes, and your partner may not like that. You obviously don't like it either, but you're necessarily caught up in your efforts to get well. The other person feels fine and wants to get on with his life. To tell the truth, what Jack

wanted was to have it like it used to be. I'm sure it can be very tempting under these circumstances to say, 'Hey, listen, I'll see you.' For someone like myself, who doesn't have a lot of job skills, that thought is devastating. And I knew he'd take the kids too. What would I have left? I'd have this horrible disease, be dependent on other people to take care of me, and my two most important things—my husband and family— would be lost."

Nat Myerson knows the experience:

"Even if there's no question that you're going to stick by the person, as I knew I was, it can get pretty rough. We were at the point that we were both falling apart and weren't much good to each other. But in a situation like that someone has to work at keeping the spirits up. Janet is a very strong person. I'm no weakling myself, but Janet has had to go through some rough times in her life. Her mother died when she was young, and her father is an alcoholic who is always getting himself into trouble. You learn to deal with that kind of thing, or it gets to you. So Janet developed this very practical approach to life— you don't let things get you down.

"The problem is that her philosophy anticipates that there will always be some way to get through the crisis. With MS there didn't seem to be any hope. I could see Janet was confused, and when I felt her sinking, I began to fall apart. I never let her know that, of course, but I really didn't know what to do. Seeing someone you love so much in such a devastating physical and emotional state . . . it's very hard to think straight. I know she was very concerned about not being able to take care of the kids—like a man would be if he couldn't work and support his family. She never even talked about not being able to go back to her job. It was just not being able to take care of the babies.

"We didn't spend much time hoping that staying in bed would help Janet's MS. She was so sick that we were ready to try anything. Like she said, our usual strategy broke down because we couldn't figure out a solution to our problem. Thank God, some other people were thinking for us. My brother heard about Dr. Soll from someone, and he told me and I told Janet. She was not impressed at first, and she didn't

want to go. I remember she said something to the effect of 'If this guy's any good, what's he doing in Iowa? I don't even know where it is.' But I told her, 'You're going, and that's it.' So she did. We had to wheel her onto the plane, and she really hated that, but my brother went with her. She couldn't have gone alone, and I was afraid that if I had gone, once we got there I wouldn't be able to leave her."

Janet continues their story.

"They put me in the hospital right away. You can imagine how much I enjoyed that, after my experiences with the hospital in Philadelphia. The first thing they wanted to do was give me another spinal. It took them two days to talk me into it, but my resistance was weakening about then, and my head was swimming. I was very, very confused. I wanted them to send me to a shrink. I work in a psychiatric school, and I figured a shrink could help me stop crying and learn how to cope.

"In reality it was good for me to go to Iowa by myself. It gave me time to think, and I needed that. I thought about all the 'what-ifs.' Because I was so afraid that the treatment I was getting wouldn't work, I tried to develop contingencies for all the problems I thought I might encounter. Being in the hospital also gave me a chance to be with other people with MS. There were some people who were in worse shape than I was, although I never would have thought that could be possible before I got there. So I saw the continuum of what multiple sclerosis can be like, and I realized that I had a chance.

"Before I went to Waterloo I couldn't do anything. I looked like a ghost because I had lived in my bed. At home, when they brought me some food, I'd try to sit up, but I usually just ended up laying my head back on the pillow and putting a spoonful of something in my mouth now and then. I knew I should eat, to keep my strength up, but I didn't really want to. My poor little Irish girl, when she had time, would help me into the shower. After I finished she'd dry me off and help me into my clothes. Actually I hardly ever wore anything but pajamas because I never got out of bed. Sometimes when a friend came by I'd make the effort to put something on and go

downstairs. A couple of times I even tried to eat at the table, but it was just easier in bed. About the only thing I could do was talk. I can always talk.

"During my first few days in Iowa I didn't get any better. They had to wheelchair me everywhere. I really didn't like that, but I wasn't in a position to argue. They even had to wheelchair me to physical therapy. They kept me there almost two weeks. Dr. Soll wanted to keep me longer, but I wouldn't stay. I wanted to get back to the kids. One day I just called Nat and told him I was coming home. He was surprised. I said, 'You just watch, I'm going to walk off that plane.' They sent my bother-in-law again—although I didn't want them to—but I was so horribly weak I probably couldn't have gotten home by myself. I did walk off the plane, however. Everything was golden from there."

Janet Myerson was lucky; she found the answer to controlling multiple sclerosis almost as soon as she was diagnosed. So did Suzanne, whose random call to the information operator paid off. Neither Suzanne nor Janet had to suffer through years of frightening symptoms with no hope of treatment or control. Cindy Morse, on the other hand, spent a year trying to do what her doctor told her. She stayed home, tried not to overdo, and took her medication when her symptoms flared up. But she never stopped hoping that there was some other way. A friend told her about the clinic in Iowa where they were successfully treating multiple sclerosis. She went back to her physician to see if he knew about it and if he would recommend her going.

Cindy recalls the incident:

"You know what he said to me? He told me he wouldn't give me his 'good grace to go out there.' I felt that I needed his permission to go so I could be reimbursed by my insurance. But it turned out it was a lost cause. He insisted the idea was 'bullshit.' I kept pressing and finally just said, 'I'm going anyway because I will try anything.' He answered, 'Well, that's the desperation of the disease. You'll probably end up in a wheelchair anyhow.'

"I was pretty sure I was going to go to Iowa before I went to

see him, but his reaction only made me more determined. It was probably my grandfather's experience haunting me, but I felt like that doctor would be waiting for me to walk in there someday with a bad exacerbation so he could say to me, 'You're not walking too well; maybe you'd better get a cane.' I know now that it's OK to use a cane, if you get into trouble and need some help to build yourself back up to where you can walk again. But I can't forget the story of my grandfather.

"So I went to Iowa and went through the program. I think the best thing about it was being with other MS patients. The treatment helped, and I learned how to take care of myself. Being with other people who have the same peculiar disease, swapping stories and experiences, can make you feel like you're not so alone. The MS patients met regularly every day. We were a small group when I was there, probably only ten or twelve patients, but we were always in each other's rooms. We talked a lot about the problems we were having at home, especially how difficult it can be to get around. We also exchanged tips and recipes, and I still do that by mail.

"When it came time to go home I was afraid to leave the hospital. I was concerned that I wouldn't be able to maintain myself on the program and I'd be back where I started from. I felt safe in the hospital because most things were taken care of for us. But I knew I couldn't stay there forever. Besides, I missed my husband and our home.

"It was spring when I left Waterloo, and I've always felt like that was a symbol of what my stay there did for me—it gave me hope for a new beginning."

Peter Samuels leans forward on his couch.

"The paradox of medicine is that it's not now, nor ever has been, an exact science. And, fascinatingly, as an organized body of knowledge, it's relatively young, which means that an individual physician can never possibly live up to the routinely predictable performance we expect of him. We should also keep in mind that the average clinician—the doctor out in practice—is not a scientist. His mission and goal are to take care of people; that's why he went to medical school. Physicians are trained to treat patients according to certain tested

and prescribed procedures. Very rarely are they encouraged to investigate disease or attempt innovative treatment. During their education, medical students learn about a host of diseases, specifically how to identify each one from their symptoms and how to apply the available range of procedures, medications, and surgeries. A few will go on to medical research, but most will become doctors who serve the public in some form of practice or another.

"The history of medicine is of trial-and-error discovery of what types of treatment work for which diseases. Crucial to this process is the understanding that there are some conditions for which nothing can be done. This, in fact, is probably one of the most alarming realizations that a physician must face—to be confronted by someone who is ill with a disease the doctor doesn't fully understand and unfortunately can't do much about. Healing the sick is not always possible. In such circumstances the physician may have little more to offer than concern and consolation.

"In this country universities and teaching hospitals have traditionally been centers for research into the causes and effects of disease, along with experimentation with new drugs and treatment techniques. So it is to these institutions that physicians and scientists who are curious about the human disease process are attracted. Such individuals push the study of medicine forward by acting on hunches and determinedly pursuing perplexing questions about what makes the human organism work, how it succumbs to illness, and how to heal it. If their research is valid and their conclusions pass muster with their peers, their discoveries may become part of the teaching curriculum of our medical schools. If they are on the right track but their findings are preliminary, they will be referred back to their institution for further work. Perhaps others will also become inspired to take up their problem.

"Because modern medicine has become very complex, today's research effort requires a substantial investment in dollars, support facilities, and personnel. The days of the independent scientist or physician laboring in his or her own lab over a life-consuming problem are virtually over. One needs

to be affiliated with a research group in a university or hospital. Aside from the obvious benefits of shared equipment and support, this system provides the serious investigator with the essential opportunity of interacting with his peers.

"Now, having delivered a lecture on the current state of medical research, I will tell you that when I realized I was not happy with the way the treatment of my disease was progressing I decided it was time to see if any effort was being undertaken that might shed some light on my affliction. As a physician with a disease medicine doesn't understand and which it currently classifies as untreatable, I decided to go back to my roots to try to find some answers. And it was there I found them. It took me longer than I had hoped, but I found them still.

"I went to the University of Minnesota medical school's multiple sclerosis clinic. First I went through the regular MS program; then I heard about this fellow who had some new kind of approach to my disease. The thing that intrigued me was that he was a physician working on a Ph.D. degree. 'Ah,' I thought to myself, 'a scientist. Maybe he has the answer.'

"Of course, it turned out that Dr. Soll didn't have 'the answer' at that exact time, but he was on the way. As I started working with him, my own professional curiosity was stimulated. I was generally intrigued by the work of the entire group with which he was associated. I began to step back from my illness and view it with the detachment of an outside observer. I allowed myself the thought that perhaps I had found my mission as a physician—to use my special skills as a doctor to verify the course of my own disease. After all those years of wallowing in self pity, working with Dr. Soll provided me with hope and inspiration and appealed to me as a professional.

"I started keeping records, observing and evaluating my symptoms, noticing changes with the treatment I was receiving. This experience served me in good stead when Dr. Soll finally got around to food allergies, because I was already practiced and comfortable at observing and recording the minutiae of everyday life. The fear of losing my wife and children

had always nagged at me, from the first day I was diagnosed with MS, but what truly motivated me was a mania against losing my sense of self. I was haunted by the demon that I would become so incapacitated that I wouldn't be able to work at the specialty for which I'd trained.

"When I think back, an additional stimulating factor about that time was the exhilaration of working hand in hand with my physician. It reminded me of the days of the family doctor with his black bag—when you could expect your physician to come by your home at any hour of the day or night and, if not diagnose and treat your illness, at least offer support and comfort. Working with Dr. Soll restored some of my original vision of the mission of medicine and reminded me that it is important for the physician to make time to listen to his patients, even if all he can return to them is a sense of warmth and concern.

"The fact that I was responsible for reporting to Dr. Soll on my behavior also influenced me. When you know you are accountable to someone, you're more motivated to do what you're supposed to do. Other MS patients have told me that they have developed similar relationships with other people in their life—a nurse, a physical therapist, a fellow MS patient, or perhaps their spouse. I found it to be important to me, and I know it's been helpful for many people. I suppose another thing that proved to be very helpful is that I received tremendous feedback from the realization that I was doing something to help myself. There was an obvious cause-and-effect relationship that I couldn't avoid when I saw the results of my actions. This can be very exhilarating and also very educational. You can't miss the obvious—if you overdo and end up with a cold or an infection, your MS symptoms get worse. As a consequence, you become a little more diligent about taking care of yourself and eating well, things like that. It keeps you on your toes."

Suzanne Baccone describes the dependence she developed because of her disease.

"I'd call Dr. Soll whenever I had a flare-up. I'd start right in describing my symptoms. Sometimes it would be something small. Other times I'd be in a panic because I couldn't see or

something like that. When I went blind for those weeks that summer, for example, that really scared me and I immediately called Dr. Soll. He listened carefully to what I had to say and then asked me about what I'd been doing with myself. Of course I had to admit that I'd been cheating—that I had sneaked a few cigarettes and had pigged out on chocolate. After a while I got tired of doing that. I have my emotions under better control now. It seems the more control you have over the MS, the more your emotions settle down. If you're not going around feeling crazy, you have the emotional energy to watch your behavior more carefully. Eating is a basic drive, after all, and people like me, when they get upset they go right for the thing they crave, and that's not good for you. Or I'd just say to myself, 'I don't care, things aren't going so well, and I know I'll feel better if I give in and have this chocolate bar.'

"When I realized how much I was calling Dr. Soll I started monitoring myself more carefully. It just took a little while for me to prove to myself that I could avoid an exacerbation by paying more attention to what I was doing and calling Dr. Soll only when I had a real emergency. I still don't keep a real strict diary and all that, but I know what I'm doing and am more responsible about it. I still worry. I'm like everyone else with MS: I want to believe that this remission will last. But I know now that I have a lot to do with keeping it that way. That feels pretty good; it eliminates some of that feeling of having a monkey on my back who can appear anytime for no apparent reason.

"I've actually found another doctor. I was so crazy for a while that I called Dr. Soll for everything—from my appendicitis to my kids' colds. I located a physican in another town close by. He's young and interested in what I'm doing and willing to work with me. I really think it's important to have a doctor you can talk to, even though I realize that the ultimate responsibility falls on me. Nobody can follow me around and constantly tell me how to behave."

Janet Myerson shouts across the swimming pool at one of the kids who's trying to get the dog to jump in with her, then continues the conversation.

"Listen, I like to swim. I also like to jog and play tennis; actually I love tennis. Anything that's going to make it possible for me to do those things, I'm going to give it a try. I mean, I thought I was going to have to spend the rest of my life in bed. Besides, all that exercise makes you look good, and everyone knows how important that is to me. I'm working on getting my jogging mileage up right now because I've got my eye on a new pair of running shoes. If I don't make two miles, Nat won't buy them for me and I'll have to shell out the cash myself.

"One of the biggest problems for people with MS, and they might not realize it initially, is the question of how the world perceives them now that they're wearing a new label—sick. You become concerned about how your family is going to react, as well as your friends and your employer. The biggest unanswered question, of course, is what do you think about yourself? I suppose a lot of people do what I did at first: go home from the hospital and go to bed. You're depressed anyway, so that's a great temptation. Isolating yourself seems to help for a while. But what you really need is support. Then you get this need for information—just to be able to talk to someone. And you can also use a pat on the back once in a while. I have a friend who's a physical therapist. He's helped me a lot. At first, when I came home from the hospital we talked. Then when I got back from Iowa we talked some more. I knew I'd have to get into a regular program because I'd been such a physical person before the attack. Before we got started, though, Ian said to me, 'Listen, if you're serious about physical therapy, you're going to have to work at it, really work. I can help, but it's your show.'

"Well that's all I had to hear. There's a way out of this thing? OK, let's do it. By that time I was watching my diet pretty well. My mother-in-law bought cases of the foods she knew I could eat. We could have opened a health food store with all the stuff she bought. But I needed that, too—the attitude of 'That's OK; we'll do whatever we can to help you work with this thing.' I know some people whose families give them hell about their diet. They complain or they tempt them. Compared to that, I had all the support in the world. But I was like a tiger once I knew there was something I could

do about this thing. Just like a tiger. Nobody was going to stop me."

Janet's big problem was the fine motor skills, but she was to become self-sufficient. The physical therapy department in the Waterloo hospital had a grab bag full of gadgets to help patients get back to doing things for themselves. Janet explains it.

"I had this gadget for zipping up my pants—nothing unusual, just a paper clip attached to the zipper. But it did the job. If I hadn't known about it, I might have been beaten by the simple task of getting dressed. A lot of people with MS make do. If they can't zip a zipper on their pants, they'll switch to wearing skirts. Well I don't like skirts that much, especially when I'm running around with the kids and all that. It really would have bothered me to have to change my way of dressing. So I just went bananas when they showed me about that little paper clip. It's a small thing, but you get the point.

"When you start to have little successes like that, then you say, 'OK, bring on the big ones.' But think what would happen if you never took the first step."

Each of these people and many others like them have made a choice. They elected not to accept what they were told about multiple sclerosis. Although they may not have been consciously aware of it at the time, when they decided to try the clinic in Iowa they became pioneers. In the true spirit of those who break new ground, they were banking on the hope that what they would find would be better than what they were leaving behind. In abandoning the safety of the established and conventional, they were risking the possibility that they might not be able to return if their new direction didn't bring them what they were seeking.

It is probably safe to say that most of them didn't give that possibility much thought. When your life is threatened by a disease like MS you probably want action, not words. In such situations emotions such as frustration and fear are strong motivators. Nonetheless, it takes courage to do what many of these people did for the first time in their life—make a decision about their health which differed from the advice and counsel of their physician.

Having made that decision, and having experienced success as a result of doing so, these people chose the next step: to continue. If you asked them why, each one will undoubtedly give you the same answer: "I stick to it because it works. I proved it with myself, and I continue to prove it every day."

3

THE MYSTERY
OF MS AND
SOME THEORIES

Multiple sclerosis is the most common disorder of the central nervous system afflicting young adults in North America and northern Europe. In the United States the National Institute of Neurological and Communicative Disorders and Stroke, the official government agency that keeps track of such things, estimates that 500,000 Americans have MS and MS-related disease.[1] Although this widespread incidence has generated increasing interest, the actual cause of multiple sclerosis remains unknown. Since it was identified in 1835, the disease has continued to intrigue and baffle researchers.[2]

At its best, medical science works in a straightforward manner—seeking to understand a disease's etiology and to identify its clinical course before attempting to develop a treatment and hopefully a cure. Accidents have occasionally happened, however. Occasionally a drug developed to treat one disease may be found to be effective with another. Or a chance event, such as knocking over a specimen jar in a laboratory, produces—in a diligent but frustrated scientist—the "aha" response that suggests another more productive approach.

Although an enormous amount of basic and clinical research has been accomplished, no substantive inroads have been made in finding a cure for MS. There are drugs available to help manage the acute attacks, and pharmaceutical technology has produced some therapies for improving and controlling complications occurring during the condition's often ruthless course.

Most simply put, multiple sclerosis is a degenerative disease of the body's central nervous system. Impulses sent along this complex network activate the gross and subtle movements that we perform thousands of times a day— from running a mile to scratching our nose. Signals move rapidly from the brain down the lines of this system, carrying messages to literally every part of the body. These nerve impulses stimulate appropriate muscle groups, and movement results. If there is some disruption of the impulse as it travels through the system—if it's interrupted in any way— the movement the brain dictates is not completed. This action is really not very different from that of common household electricity traveling from a source of energy along an electric wire to an appliance. If you turn on a light, for example, and there is a short in the line, the energy you activated when you pressed the switch will not reach the light. You will be left in the dark, trying to navigate back to your room balancing your midnight snack.

The nerve fibers that comprise the central nervous system are coated with a fatty protein material called *myelin,* somewhat in the same way an electrical wire is protected by insulation. In the MS-affected body the myelin surrounding the nerve fibers is randomly destroyed. This has the same effect as a short in an electrical line; it interferes with the transmission of signals—from the brain to the fingers, or the feet, or the left arm, or the bladder. The designated movement either is not executed or is executed in a faulty manner. The loss of the myelin from the white matter in the brain and spinal cord encompasses a sharply demarcated area that looks much like an inkblot and leaves behind a firmer, rubbery texture to the tissue. These areas are referred to as *multiple sclerosis plaques.*

For the most part these plaques still contain intact nerve fibers, but they are stripped of their myelin. Some MS patients fear that once an area is robbed of these vital cells of the myelin the damage is permanent, meaning that symptoms typical of "short circuits" will persist. Curiously, however, function has been seen to return even though obvious plaques are still present. The scientific explanation for this process goes something like this: Cells, called *oligodendrocytes,* are lined up and down the long nerve fibers, predominantly in the white matter, and literally wrap their membranes around the nerve fibers. During an attack of MS these cells are destroyed. For practical purposes this results in the breakup or degeneration of the myelin protein. Thus, it is not correct to speak of degenerative changes in myelin, per se, but of the death of the specialized nerve cells, or oligodendrocytes, that compose the myelin.

The general effect of the breakdown in the myelin covering of the nerve fibers is to influence the speed and efficiency of nerve impulses. A significant slowing of the rate at which impulses travel throughout the body will obviously impair normal movement such as walking. Likewise, a complete block of the impulse can also occur. Either of these reactions causes the symptoms we usually associate with MS. Bodily functions go haywire because messages either don't reach their destination or are delayed. Aside from the primary symptoms experienced by the MS patient, there can be secondary complications resulting from this failure in signal transmission. If a person loses bladder control, for example, and doesn't know when he has to void, the effect can be to leave a residual amount of urine in the bladder. Stagnation then causes an increased susceptibility to urinary tract infection. As we shall see, an infection in turn can precipitate an exacerbation of multiple sclerosis.

The clinical manifestations of MS vary with the location and extent of the plaques in the central nervous system. Often one of the first symptoms is blurred vision or temporary blindness. Dizziness, unsteadiness, or tremors in the arms and legs also might occur. Sometimes the first symptom is numbness in an arm or leg. Weakness or paralysis of an extremity also might appear early and cause difficulty in walking, from dragging a foot to the buckling of a knee under the person's weight. To the MS sufferer the meaning of these symptoms is obvious. Others may watch helplessly as a relative or friend struggles to move a leg forward, lift a package, or dress or feed himself—any of the hundreds of little things that make an individual self-sufficient and give life significance.

If the nerves in the spinal cord are affected, symptoms are usually focused in the extremities or trunk of the body rather than in the head and neck. This can produce difficulty of movement and can also result in loss of sensation or bodily functions such as bladder and bowel control. If the MS lesions appear in the brain, symptoms can also include weakness or numbness, dizziness, unsteadiness, and problems with coordination such as slurred speech patterns or visual loss. Jerking eye movement usually results from involvement of the brain stem, the connecting area between the brain and spinal cord.

The multiple sclerosis patient doesn't live with the constant fear of death, as is often the case with other diseases we don't understand, such as the various forms of cancer. Nor is there the persistent drag of physical pain as in other chronic illnesses like arthritis. Instead, the individual with MS is saddled with the demoralizing apprehension that his disease may become worse. He lives with the fear that the next attack will not only bring immediate incapacitation, but may also result in such comprehensive damage that recovery will be impossible. In this aspect MS can be the most cruel of all diseases because it strikes people during the prime of life— usually between their twenties and forties. It is the time when most of us are just beginning to live in the adult sense. Goals are being established, a profession is selected, perhaps a partner has been chosen. Likely as not, the individual is far from accomplishing what he envisions for himself.

MS can leave those it afflicts with an unsatisfied hunger for experience and achievement. Without proper therapy, the physical incapacitation of the disease can literally slow down an individual to the point of being housebound. The most fundamental physical danger from MS is that involvement can become so widespread that functions necessary for self-care will fail, so that the long-term result can be total dependency. Also, the emotional effects of suffering with a condition that seems to be impossible to treat can destroy an individual's motivation, such that he slowly reduces activity, doing less and less for himself, and finally succumbs to the symptoms of the disease.

It is true that many MS patients don't require the wheelchairs and canes most of us associate with the disease. Some are only minimally incapacitated. Others suffer recurrent attacks of varying symptoms, from temporary blindness to paralysis. Still, there are other individuals who unfortunately slip slowly and resolutely downhill. Because of the disease's erratic patterns, many individuals may escape diagnosis. This variation in symptoms, along with inconsistency in diagnosis, makes our efforts to investigate and understand multiple sclerosis extremely difficult. Such complications thwart the usual strategy of medical research—the controlled, double-blind study—which would enable us to verify attempts at treatment and cure.

Amid the steady work and recurrent confusion associated with the study of multiple sclerosis, three principal theories have emerged, none of which has been conclusively proven, but each of which contains elements that shed some light on the disease. We will refer to these three theories as:

(1) the Viral Theory;
(2) the Autoimmune Theory; and
(3) the Composite Theory.

As is usual in scientific work of this type, elaborate rationales have been developed to identify each of these theoretical approaches as distinct from the other and thus justify an experimental and clinical direction. Such activity results from the friendly competition existing among researchers who must necessarily focus on specific aspects of a problem. This arrangement is generally considered effective, although combining more than one approach has also been known to produce an occasional "aha" that can lead to a breakthrough in understanding a perplexing disease. In fact, as we shall see, something like this seems to be happening with MS.

The Viral Theory was the first to be considered. Most simply put, it holds that multiple sclerosis results from a specific viral infection. In this regard, the most likely culprit is considered to be either a slow-acting virus or the body's delayed reaction to a specific virus such as measles. The second possible explanation for MS, the Autoimmune Theory, proposes some form of autoimmune reaction in which the body mistakenly attacks its own tissues. A similar malfunction of the immune system system has also been implicated in other degenerative diseases such as arthritis and rheumatic fever. The third explanation, the Composite Theory, suggests that MS is the result of a combination of these two mechanisms so that the body becomes confused in the presence of a new or unknown virus and in some way activates its immune system against itself.

To understand and evaluate each of these three suggested explanations we must first understand the elements involved, primary of which is the body's system for protecting itself against disease. The body's immune system is a complicated and awe-inspiring piece of machinery, the complexity of which we are just beginning to comprehend. To execute its defenses, the immune system must first develop self-recognition so that it can verify that the body has been invaded by a disease-producing substance—what scientists call an *antigen.* This crucial ability to distinguish between its own cells and tissues and any nonbody substances such as a virus, pollen, or chemical normally occurs very early in life. Without this capability, we would be defenseless.

Once the agents of the immunological system have determined that the body has been invaded, they set to work against the potential troublemaker. In these battles against irritating or disease-producing antigens one of the primary weapons is antibodies, proteins produced within the body, which combine with the potentially toxic invaders to neutralize and incapacitate them. Antibodies are one of our first lines of defense and produce what is referred to as *humoral immunity.* This means that antibodies to specific substances are present in our blood and tissues, in all our secretions, and are constantly available to react against intruding foreign substances.

One of the excellent characteristics of our immune system is that it has a memory. If the body is again invaded by the same threatening substance, the initial identification process can be shortened, and the production of the appropriate antibodies will begin much more quickly.

As scientists have studied the immune system and have come to understand the antigen-antibody relationship, they have been able to encourage this natural process and develop a safer method of protection against infectious disease. We experience this very early in life as the unpleasant vaccination "shot" from our family doctor. Until vaccination, or inoculation, became a widespread practice in this country, death and illness from bacterial or viral infections that produced such diseases as typhoid, polio, and smallpox were a very serious health problem. In vaccination, either a milder or an inactivated form of the disease is injected into the individual and the body obliges by tooling up to get rid of the foreign invader, creating the necessary antibodies to fight it. The individual never actually "comes down" with the disease, but if he were to come in contact with it again, his system would "remember" it and summon up antibody protection. If the inoculation is successful, the individual is said to "be immune" to that specific infection. This doesn't mean that he is completely protected from "catching" the disease, but that his body "knows" how to fight it and will want to rid itself of it before it can cause substantial damage.

Given this process, it would indeed seem logical to consider that MS could result from an invading virus to which the individual hasn't yet become immune. The course of action then would be to develop an antiviral vaccine that could be used to control multiple sclerosis, just as vaccination has controlled other viral-induced illnesses.

THE VIRAL THEORY

The Viral Theory is supported by the fact that MS seems to occur more frequently in certain parts of the world and is relatively nonexistent in others. Northern climates, for example, seem to produce a considerably higher incidence of the disease. It may also be that higher risk is associated with inadvertent exposure to an environmental agent in a more northern climate before the individual turns fifteen. This has been suspected because it appears that a person who moves south from a northerly area after that age carries with him the same likelihood of contracting MS as if he had not moved. This particular age relationship could also suggest an effect from the normal hormonal changes associated with the onset of puberty.

For many years epidemiological studies have contributed to an increased understanding of MS. As we said, it is now well known that the incidence of MS is higher in more northern latitudes of the United States and Europe compared to corresponding southern areas. Studies show that the highest incidence of multiple sclerosis is located in the Orkney and Shetland Islands, relatively isolated islands off the north coast of Scotland. Here there seems to be particular concern for cleanliness and sanitation, which may mean that the inhabitants are not exposed to as many childhood viruses as in other places and are thus limited in the range of diseases to which they might be immune. Some recent and interesting epidemiological work comes from the Faeroe Islands, where an epidemic of multiple sclerosis occurred between 1943 and 1960. The outbreak appears to be related to the arrival of British troops during World War II and suggests the possibility of an infection from a virus with a long incubation period.[3] Such a virus might gain access to the body, remain unidentified by the immunological system, spread uninhibitedly to an isolated area like the brain, and appear at a later date.

Considerable research has been devoted to attempts to identify naturally occurring viruses capable of selectively involving the central nervous system. Infections such as rubeola (red measles) and rubella (three-day measles) have been found to persist in the central nervous systems of some individuals. Such viruses may exist quietly within the nervous system for a number of years and then, for some still unknown reason, produce inflammation that leads to a progressive deterioration of neurological function. The rubeola virus can cause a condition called *subacute sclerosing panencephalitis*, while the rubella virus, or three-day measles, is responsible for a condition called *progressive panencephalitis*. Research has focused particularly on possible mechanisms for persistence of viruses in the body's tissues, as well as why renewed inflammation begins after a period of latent activity. Although few conclusive results have materialized from such studies, it is thought that because these and other similar conditions exist, it is possible that a similar virus might be responsible for MS.

Assuming that a virus does cause MS, it would indeed be logical to suggest that it would have to be one of those that selectively inhabit the central nervous system. Herein lies one of the difficulties with an exclusively viral theory for MS. Typically those viruses that show a preference for the nervous system search out the nerve tissue itself. In multiple sclerosis, however, a remarkable preservation of the axon—the part of the nerve cell through which the impulse travels—remains, even when the myelin sheath is missing. The selective destruction of myelin cells would seem to suggest that a virus causing MS would have to have a particular affinity for some parts of the specialized cell membranes from which myelin is formed and not other types of cells that constitute nerve tissue. Unfortunately, most viruses that attack the nervous system demonstrate just the opposite behavior. On the other hand, it is interesting to note that certain mutant viruses found in mice now have been shown to infect the myelin cells.[4] So this may be a promising avenue after all, despite the fact that up to this time recurrent attempts to isolate a specific virus in the tissues of MS patients have proven unsuccessful.

It is also important to remember that one reason the nerve fibers survive the white blood cell attack may be that the nerve cell bodies from which nerve fibers extend are removed from the area of inflammation involving the myelin. Although the nerve fibers are literally skinned of their myelin coating at particular areas of inflammation, they, themselves, receive sustenance from the nerve cell body. This source of nourishment means that there is a flow of cytoplasm and other essential nutrients down through the axon of the nerve cells. The myelin cells, on the other hand, are very small and completely dependent on the local blood supply for their sustenance. All of which is to say that the nerve cells are sufficiently far from the point of inflammation caused by the reaction against the myelin that they don't seem to be affected by the resulting inflammation and destruction and can continue about their business.

Numerous variations of the Viral Theory have been suggested. The first hypothesis is that the individual comes into contact with what is called a *slow virus.* Such a virus grows slowly but steadily in the body, with the result that it takes a long time for the immunological sensors to recognize it. We also know that there are dormant viruses that can lie quietly in the human organism for years, only to become activated at some later date, triggered by their own activity or some as yet unknown phenomenon. There are difficulties with the concept of a slow virus causing MS, however, in that only a few types of slow viruses have been identified in humans, and their clinical course is one of increasing disability at a slow and predictable pace, with the eventual outcome of death. This usually occurs a year after the clinical manifestation of symptoms, as in Creutzfeldt-Jakob disease.

THE AUTOIMMUNE THEORY

The possibilities of the Viral Theory aside, other researchers have produced some interesting work on the immune system that supports the possibility of an Autoimmune Theory for multiple sclerosis. To explain their thoughts we have to meet another member of the immunological team, the white blood cells. There are several types of white blood cells, some of which actually produce antibodies. Other white blood cells function differently, producing what we call *cell-mediated,* as opposed to antibody or humoral, *immunity.* The white blood cells are found throughout the body's tissues and fluids. While antibodies are ubiquitous, reacting with specific foreign substances whenever they come in contact with them, the white blood cells seek out foreign invaders by infiltrating contaminated tissues and directly attacking the virus or bacteria. They may also help synthesize antibodies at the site. Like the other agents of the immune system, some specialized white blood cells have a memory and will immediately react if the body subsequently experiences a similar attack. So efficient is the action of the white blood cells that at times it has been necessary to cut it off, as in organ transplantation, where the immune system may classify the donated organ as foreign and attempt to reject it.

To further consider the Autoimmune Theory of MS one has to review a number of additional factors. Remember that the body's recognition of self occurs early in life, at the time of birth or immediately thereafter. But some parts of the body may not be fully developed by that time or are isolated from the rest of body, making them vulnerable to attack as foreign. For example, myelin in the brain and spinal cord develops late in humans. Myelinization typically doesn't begin until the later part of fetal life or the early period of neonatal life and generally is not completed until the child begins walking. The Autoimmune argument thus maintains that the mature immunological system won't recognize myelin as self because it just wasn't around and accessible when the body was developing self-recognition.[5]

A second factor to be considered in support of the Autoimmune Theory for MS is that some type of problem may exist in the action of the white blood cells of MS patients. This area of research has opened up a tremendous field of investigation concerning the manner in which the white blood cells are regulated and how they function. It has also identified a wide variety of different types of these cells, thus permitting a much better understanding of these components of the immune system.

To better understand the relevant aspects of research involving the white blood cells requires an awareness of their function. Two major groups of white blood cells comprise the immune system. These are the B-cells and the T-cells. B-cells produce antibodies of different types, sometimes independently and sometimes with the assistance of T-cells. Antibodies may be compared to bullets with which the body fights the enemy, whereas the T-cells would be more properly characterized as soldiers fighting with bayonets. For this reason, the T-cells are related to the cell-mediated immune reaction. The T-cells can in turn be divided into three types: the Helper T-cells, the suppressor T-cells and the Killer T-cells. The Helper Ts aid the B-cells in producing an effective antibody response to foreign antigens. Suppressor Ts, on the other hand, depress a variety of immune reactions. In so doing, they tend to keep the immune system in check or under control. The Killer T-cells, sometimes called K-cells, are cytotoxic, or destructive, to the specific cells they attack. A predictable target for their action might be a cell infected by a virus, a tumor cell, or a cell from a transplanted organ or bacteria.

In the typical immunological reaction involving white blood cells, certain cells, the Helper and Killer Ts, are activated and get right to fighting the infection. Suppressor T-cells then slow down the defensive reaction after the threat has been mastered, in effect turning off the defenses. Obviously the correct balance among the various types of white blood cells is necessary if the immune system is to function correctly. If this balance is tipped somehow, the affected individual may end up at risk from an agent his immune system doesn't want to fight or, even worse, with an overreaction that theoretically could turn his body against itself.

In this regard researchers at Scripps Institute have found that during an exacerbation an MS patient may demonstrate only a 6-percent presence of suppressor T-cells, while at other times the percentage will rise to as much as 17 percent. This contrasts to non-MS patients whose percentage of suppressor cells routinely runs to about 12 percent of their white blood cell count.[6] Another study produced the finding that during acute attacks of MS suppressor T-cell activity is reduced. In fact, in some cases reduced suppressor T-cell activity was found to be present even before the attack began.[7] This has enhanced speculation that exacerbations of

MS may result from reduced suppressor T-cells, which thus would permit overreactivity of the other components of the immune system such as the K-cells. It has also been suggested that these suppressor cells might be the object of a simultaneous attack against themselves and the myelin antigen in the central nervous system.

Thus, the idea of an Autoimmune Theory for MS is a plausible explanation, provided we could identify the exact nature of the malfunction of the immune system and the mechanism by which its agents, the white blood cells, come in contact with the central nervous system. These possibilities, along with the Composite Theory, will be explored in the following chapter.

4

THE ROLE OF
THE IMMUNE SYSTEM
IN MS

For as long as man has been thinking he has expended time and energy pondering the meaning of life. Philosophers have spent endless hours seeking answers to two ever-perplexing questions: "Why are we here, and what are we supposed to be doing with ourselves?" Warriors and kings have evoked the blessing of God and country, not necessarily in that order. Poets have observed our efforts to civilize the world and have suggested a few things we can do with our efforts.

In modern times—relatively speaking—a new voice has emerged, and it belongs to the scientist. If, for example, you were to ask an immunologist for his opinion of life, he might tell you that the process we call living amounts to a constant struggle between ourselves and our environment. His is a view of a battle constantly being waged between our immune system and the wide range of potentially dangerous substances to which we are routinely exposed. Without the immune system, everyone from poets to kings would find it difficult to survive.

We have indicated that close behind the Viral Theory for MS have come some thoughts about a possible involvement of the immune system. To evaluate an autoimmune explanation, we must consider ways in which the immune system can malfunction. This actually isn't such an unusual occurrence; in fact, one of the most common breakdowns in the human immune system is a condition many of us live with all our lives—allergy.

You, or someone you know, may be all too familiar with the symptoms of hay fever or have an irritating reaction to dust, grass, or any of the hundreds of common allergens that have been identified. Someone who considers strolling through a flowering field in the springtime an exercise in masochism, rather than an uplifting aesthetic experience, undoubtedly suffers from problems in his immune system. Such breakdowns cause innately nonirritating substances to produce a range of uncomfortable symptoms.

While each of us is sensitive in varying degrees to the same or similar substances that might trigger our immune system, some people discover they are supersensitive—to pollen, for example. This causes the overproduction of antibodies called *reagins* and the condition we know as hay fever. Because the antibodies which the body activates to neutralize the effects of inhaled pollen or dust will circulate throughout one's system, this type of supersensitive response can produce uncomfortable symptoms, often requiring treatment or medication. Thus, we have the familiar allergy test and its companion, the allergy shot. We can't stop the body from becoming overly sensitive to something, but we can relieve our symptoms to that sensitivity by suppressing the action of our immunological agents.

The scientific name for this type of reaction is *immediate hypersensitivity*. Simply put, it means that the body's activation of its defense system occurs immediately upon contact with the offending substance. Such an immediate hypersensitive reaction involves humoral immunity, which depends on the action of antibodies. There is a second type of hypersensitive reaction, however, in which the immune system delays its response. When it finally does act, it calls on the additional strength of the white blood cells. This *delayed hypersensitive* reaction usually happens when the foreign substance is an infection or a transplanted organ or a tumor and has had time to establish a foothold in the body. A reaction to tuberculosis is a well known example of a delayed hypersensitive reaction.

Although science is not completely clear on the relationship of the immediate and delayed hypersensitive reactions, it appears that they both result from a combination of factors, including genetics, environment, and the age at which an individual is exposed to the irritating substance. It is not unusual for a person to have repeated exposure to a variety of potential irritants in his environment. The frequency and amount of exposure to a substance also plays a role in the ultimate development and manner in which an allergy is manifested. The immune system, like the rest of us, is usually in top form in a younger body, when it hasn't been fatigued by its constant battle against a range of foreign substances.

Although most immediate hypersensitive responses can readily be controlled by medication to suppress the action of the antibodies, delayed hypersensitivity is another matter, and hence its significance in MS. Delayed hypersensitivity involves a more primitive and longer-lasting reaction. The delayed response is one of hand-to-hand combat between our cell-mediated white blood cell defenses, specifically the Killer T-cells, and the dangerous intruder. One result of this confrontation can be irritation and damage of the very cells and tissues the body wishes to protect.

THE COMPOSITE THEORY

What has all of this to do with MS? It makes it possible for us to suggest the third explanation, the Composite Theory, for the origin and symptoms of multiple sclerosis.[1] Consider, for a moment, that a person is exposed to a measles virus. For some reason he hasn't "had" measles before. His body takes a while to activate its immunological sensors, and in the meantime the virus goes to work infiltrating cells and multiplying. It moves into all the small nooks and spaces of the body. By this time the white blood cells need help controlling the invader, and more are called in to aid in synthesizing antibodies and to attack the virus. The problem is that, having dragged its feet and allowed the virus to multiply, the immune system has a much bigger job ahead of it.

The first logical question to be asked is why didn't the body recognize the virus as a potential threat in the first place? One possibility is that perhaps the virus was so minimally irritating that its presence wasn't detected until its sheer numbers forced notice. Or perhaps this individual wasn't exposed to that particular virus as a child—either because of the geographical area in which he grew up or due to the type of sanitary conditions under which he was reared. He therefore wouldn't have developed postinfectious immunity, which involves that all-important "memory" of the white blood cells.

The fact that an individual might not have been exposed to the virus in childhood, at a time when his body was best equipped to handle it, would indicate the possibility of a more intense reaction as an adult. The younger we are when we are first exposed to a virus, the more likely it is that our body will be able to get it under control and establish permanent immunity. The diseases of childhood, such as mumps, generally come and go in children's lives without problems and usually result in a lifetime of immunity. However, an adult who somehow missed the mumps as a child and comes down with them as an adult could experience complications such as sterility, pancreatitis, or perhaps even encephalitis. Additionally, these complications mean that the situation already has resulted in the more serious consequences of a cell-mediated, delayed hypersensitive reaction. It is then too late for the humoral immunity system's antibodies to do the job adequately, so the white blood cells are needed to continue to try to discharge the intruder.

As the sensitized white blood cells react with the virus, pursuing it into the bloodstream and into the muscles, the organs, and even the very smallest spaces in the body, the result is not only damage to the tissues in the areas of combat, but a situation in which the white blood cells can find themselves in areas of the body not normally accessible to them. Thus, such a virus, traveling throughout an individual's system, might generate enough numbers so that many slip into the central nervous system, an excursion that would not ordinarily be possible. In this instance, however, its own large numbers and those of the white blood cells assault each other within the normal barrier that protects the central nervous system. Here the trouble begins.

First, the white blood cells do their work attacking the virus, which results in no small amount of damage and disarray, enhancing the tissue inflammation from the viral infection. In this heightened state of activity the white blood cells discover the myelin protein in the brain and spinal cord, to which they have not previously been exposed. Unequipped to recognize it as part of the body, and geared up for their fight against the virus, they attack the myelin as foreign.

And so, a virus that is not recognized soon enough becomes the triggering mechanism for an autoimmune reaction, specifically to the myelin, which apparently the body hasn't seen before. It is important to understand that this reaction occurs within the brain and spinal cord and the blood vessels supplying these structures. Thus, it is to these areas that the white blood cells rush for their fight.

Fundamentally, the nervous system exists in isolation. It is separated from the rest of the body by a series of semipermeable cellular membranes that selectively filter out substances attempting to gain access to it. The blood-brain barrier system, as it has been called, was first identified with the injection of dyes that routinely stain but do not damage tissues in virtually all the organs of the body. It is very difficult, however, to observe such staining in the central nervous system. This indicates that the blood-brain barrier is probably very dense under normal circumstances, which makes it usually quite effective in keeping out bacteria and viruses. Very rarely, for example, do we see an abscess develop in the brain or spinal cord. Ordinarily, when an individual becomes acutely ill with a systemic infection, the nervous system remains intact and functioning reasonably well. Someone who becomes delirious, however, would probably be suffering a breakdown in the blood-brain barrier system.

Although the barrier does a good job of keeping out bacteria and yeast and fungus infections, it appears not to be as effective against viruses. Because of their size and chemical composition, viruses tend to cross the barrier more easily, especially in large numbers. If an individual were housing a virus for the period of time it takes to multiply and move from cell to cell and organ to organ through the bloodstream, it would be logical to assume that the virus would travel into the nervous system, especially if the body had not yet recognized its presence. When the body does finally decide to put up a fight, the white blood cells it activates would necessarily follow the virus, crossing the blood-brain barrier. This is because the relative impermeability of this barrier would be affected if it were assaulted by hordes of viruses and white blood cells.

The resulting myelin-white blood cell confrontation that might occur is the phenomenon of autoimmunity. Through the preceding series of incidents, the individual becomes sensitized to his own myelin—although at this stage, the sensitivity is of a low magnitude. As we shall see, however, these circumstances set the stage for subsequent manifestations of the disease.

As this individual proceeds through life, he will experience numerous occasions in which his body struggles against potentially irritating environmental agents. Growing older, he may undergo more infections and allergic reactions. Combatting these infections and mediating these allergies produce a cumulative effect on his immune system. Eventually he may reach a stage where his original latent allergy to myelin blossoms and symptoms of multiple sclerosis appear. There have just been too many occasions of contact between his white blood cells and the antigenic substance in myelin. Although previous viral infections or allergies may not have been full-blown reactions, his body can no longer cope effectively. Thus, his subclinical allergy to myelin erupts as multiple sclerosis.

At this point it may be useful to recap what we've discussed so far. This confusion in the immune system, whereby it is unable to distinguish itself from outside substances, means that a person can literally become allergic to the cells and tissues of his own body. In this case we are concerned with certain constituents of the cells forming the myelin that line the nerve fibers in the central nervous system. Theoretically, the immune system reacts to these substances as nonself. We have seen that the likely agent that introduces the white blood cells to the myelin protein is a virus.

It is probably unreasonable to assume that an individual would often be exposed to this level of viral infection, and if this were the only factor involved, it might be that he would not again suffer another attack of MS. The clinical course of the disease, however, suggests another thought.

It is readily observed clinically that MS becomes worse in the presence of an infection and that controlling infection can decrease an exacerbation of the disease.[2] People entering treatment who can hardly walk or can't see experience a decrease in their symptoms if they are simply given antibiotics to control, for example, a clandestine bladder or respiratory tract infection.

To account for the recurrent attacks typical of MS, our Composite Theory must consider two other elements. These are *endotoxin* and the *Shwartzman reaction*. Endotoxin is a powerful, toxic substance found in the walls of the bacterial cells and released when those cells die. It is present in disease-producing bacteria of the sort that cause diarrhea or a bladder infection. This type of bacterial cell also usually inhabits the human intestinal tract. The interaction between the endotoxin released when bacteria die and the white blood cells called out to fight an infection produces the condition we know as fever.

During a bacterial infection such as an earache or tonsillitis endotoxin is released into the bloodstream, where it circulates and causes the superficial blood vessels to contract. This means that heat constantly being generated in the body by normal metabolism is trapped because it can't reach the skin through its normal avenue. Fever, therefore, is not the body's reaction to fighting an infection, as is normally assumed, but rather a reaction caused in part by endotoxin released from infectious bacteria. Humans and animals alike are extremely sensitive to endotoxin, a sensitivity that is usually acquired early in life.

As well as resulting from infection, endotoxin from very large numbers of bacteria is also naturally present in the intestines of humans as a by-product of the digestive process. If, for some reason, there were to be an irritation of the lining of the intestinal wall, causing it to become inflamed and weakening its ability to block entrance to endotoxin, minute amounts of this potent toxin could be absorbed and even slip into the body's general circulation. Since the primary business of the intestines is digestion, it follows that a prime suspect for causing irritation of the bowel might be food, especially foods an individual finds difficult to digest. Someone routinely consuming food to which he is allergic might then experience the same endotoxic effect in himself as if he were suffering from a bacterial infection.

To illustrate one of the more well-known effects of the action of endotoxin on the body, let's look at a common laboratory animal, the rabbit. If we were to administer endotoxin to a rabbit, its action would be immediately observable in the animal's ears, the site at which it typically loses body heat through the dilation of blood vessels. Before the injection of endotoxin the rabbit's ears would feel warm because of the escaping heat. A few minutes after it receives the endotoxin, however, the rabbit's ears would feel cold. As in humans, the endotoxin would cause the constriction of the surface blood vessels that transmit body heat. The animal's temperature would start to rise, just as ours would if we were experiencing the release of endotoxin from an infection.

The heat lost from the body begins to equal the heat generated, which produces a new body temperature and the reaction we've identified as fever. Endotoxin is extremely important to our discussion of multiple sclerosis because its release can enhance the action of white blood cells in combating foreign substances. An individual who has developed a sensitivity to his own myelin protein through the encounter between his white blood cells and a virus or other antigen would experience an enhancement of that reaction if endotoxin were present in the bloodstream. Such a release could result from a bladder or respiratory tract infection or from the bacteria in an inflamed intestinal wall. Thus, a latent allergy to myelin, initiated by the immune system's pursuit of a virus into the central nervous system, could blossom into a full-blown clinical reaction.

Allergic reactions to food have begun to concern scientists and physicians. Initially the idea that an intolerant reaction to food might be related to such diseases as hypertension, cancer, or atherosclerosis was met with amused silence among medical specialists. One of the reasons for this is that it's difficult to explain food allergies with standard laboratory studies or skin tests. On the other hand, the family practitioner has always been aware that certain people may have trouble digesting particular foods. Such reactions, however, have often been classified as a result of the innately irritating nature of the foods themselves interfering with a person's digestion, rather than an individual susceptibility to specific foods.

A number of clinicians and researchers have explored the possible relationship between multiple sclerosis and diet. One result has been the development of curious types of food regimens that have been applied with various levels of success. For the most part these diets have been based on the proposition that a particular food or food type causes the problem—fat has recurrently been thought to be a culprit, for example. On the other hand, it also seems to be a reasonable possibility that there may be certain foods that an individual might find intolerable on an allergic basis.

A tremendous variety of foods can be consumed in a lifetime. Repeated exposure to specific foods might result in the development of either a delayed or an immediate hypersensitivity to those foods or their by-products. The result of such a situation would be that the ingestion of a particular allergy-producing food would cause a low-grade inflammation of the intestinal wall. In turn, this would reduce the effectiveness of the wall as a barrier against both the absorption of food and the endotoxin, which is a by-product of the breakdown of bacteria. An individual with food allergies thus would be susceptible to inflammation of the intestinal wall and the decreased effectiveness of the body's primary barrier against the rather lethal effects of endotoxin.

Briefly, let us recap our proposed Composite Theory for MS. We have suggested that multiple sclerosis is initiated with a delayed hypersensitive reaction against the myelin in the central nervous system. This amounts to the body becoming allergic to its own tissues. A delayed hypersensitive reaction against myelin is triggered by a viral infection— any viral infection—which is in turn dependent on the individual's ability to respond to the virus, as well as his ability to react to the foreign nature of the myelin. In evaluating an exclusively viral theory for MS, we have to consider that it would seem reasonable to expect that steroid hormones (prednisone or ACTH) and other forms of immunosuppressive therapy, which slow down or completely inhibit the reaction of the white blood cells, would aggravate virally induced MS by allowing the viral infection to accelerate. Rather, it appears that the administration of such treatment usually has a beneficial effect in inhibiting acute exacerbations of multiple sclerosis. Additionally, it is difficult to reconcile the exacerbating and remitting course of the disease with the progressive deterioration that is common with a chronic viral infection.

However, if a viral infection were the primary cause of multiple sclerosis, a delayed hypersensitive reaction to the invading virus would contribute significantly to the damage inflicted on the nervous system. Age is obviously a factor in this reaction. The older the body, the less efficient the immune system. This has the effect of allowing the virus more time to obtain a foothold, as it incubates itself in the cells and multiplies. The more viruses generated, the more white blood cells will be needed to control the infection, and the more havoc will be created when the two clash.

The battle between the white blood cells and the foreign substance causes inflammation and tissue damage. If the virus has had sufficient time to multiply, it will circulate to all areas of the body, including the brain and nervous system. The white blood cells follow, and in the process of fighting the virus, inflammation and damage to the nervous system occur. The white blood cells thus become exposed and presumably sensitized to the myelin in the central nervous system, which they haven't seen before.

In this way the viral infection that ignites the sensitivity to myelin is like a spark that will require additional fuel before it rages into a fire. In MS the spark can die when there aren't enough potential aggravating factors to ignite the fire and keep it burning. It may take many years for the young adult to register enough allergies and infections to catalyze the underlying delayed hypersensitivity to myelin. But once the initial attack of MS appears, repeated infection and allergic reactions from food and other antigenic substances can allow the entrance of endotoxin into the body. This combines with the previously sensitized white blood cells to cause an exacerbation of the disease.

With the realization that foods to which one is sensitized may be causing a chronic and continuous absorption of endotoxin from the gut, it is possible to understand the slowly progressive nature of MS, even without the potentially destructive effects of recurrent, acute exacerbations.

The significance of these theoretical considerations is the subject of subsequent chapters.

5

FOOD ALLERGIES—
ANOTHER LINK

Los Angeles is a fashionable town. Fads—from what to wear to where to live—come and go faster than Maseratis on the freeways at 2 A.M. Reality in LA basks in the rosy glow of the seductive southern California climate and reflects the glamorous images created by its entertainment industries. People live through their senses, an enterprise that turns out to be surprisingly effective.

It would be unusual in this kind of environment not to find a reasonable number of what are generally referred to as "fine" restaurants, serving some version or another of continental cuisine and making pretentions toward consummate service. In a place like Los Angeles intentions often count more than achievement, which makes for a great deal of competition among the well-meaning. For example, a recently observed dining innovation goes something like this: The captain appears at your table to discuss your dinner. The food for the evening established, he then surprises you with an unexpected question, "Are there any food allergies?" The expression on most people's faces seems to reflect the opinion that this matter should be left to themselves and their physicians. The initial surprise passes, however, as the diners casually gaze around the table, checking with each other. The answer usually comes as a unanimous shrug of the shoulders and an offhanded "No." An occasional enterprising soul will add something ambiguous like "Not that I know of," against the possibility that the establishment might serve him something he doesn't like.

Pretensions aside, this is actually not such an inappropriate question. Food allergies, whether known and ignored or as yet undiscovered and untreated, are capable of spoiling even the most carefully planned and well-executed meal. Let's hope, however, that a well-meaning concern doesn't become a meaningless ploy. Food allergies have had enough of a bad rap without becoming fashionable.

The concept that an individual may suffer from an allergic reaction to food is still viewed with skepticism by the medical establishment, which maintains that we don't yet have the expertise to diagnose such conditions effectively. Nonetheless, the discovery of an adverse reaction to a food, a food additive, or the by-products of digestion, combined with a plan to avoid the irritating substance, have helped many people for whom established techniques of treatment could provide little relief.

Allergy—the overreaction of the body to something that is basically benign—has been an established medical fact for almost a century. The symptoms of classical allergy fall into two major categories: (1) problems in the respiratory tract such as difficulty in breathing, sneezing, runny nose, and sore throat; and (2) skin reactions, from hives to intense, disfiguring swelling. The substances that induce these reactions have become common knowledge, so that we don't blink an eye if someone says he or she is allergic to pollen, dust, mold, or even some type of chemical.[1]

Some symptoms of food allergy are often identical to other allergic reactions. However, they can also masquerade as problems in the digestive tract, including colitis, diarrhea, constipation, and chronic indigestion. Allergies to food have also been known to cause headaches, dizziness, and chronic fatigue—conditions that are often unresponsive to conventional treatment. Individual susceptibility to foodstuffs and/ or the by-products of digestion has been studied for almost as long as we've known about allergies, although the condition has not typically interested conventional allergists because of the difficulty in directly relating symptoms to the ingestion of a particular food. Also, who would expect that our favorite foods or foods we consider to be healthy could cause adverse symptoms? In response to a growing awareness of this phenomenon, as well as an increase in illness related to environmental contamination, a new area of specialization has emerged. Thanks to meticulous work, clinical ecology has been able to offer patients relief from chronic, previously untreatable symptoms.[2]

One food allergy pioneer claims that most people have difficulty tolerating one food or another, the primary problems being with eggs, wheat, corn, milk, sugar, chocolate, and nuts. Other common allergies include reactions to white potatoes, red meat, oranges, tomatoes, and bananas.[3] That so many of us may experience difficulty digesting what may even be our favorite food doesn't seem so startling when you consider that perhaps as much as half of the United States population is affected by one kind of allergy or another—many of which require treatment.

Standard medical treatment consists of controlling the allergic reaction through desensitization, a method of injecting the individual with a less potent form of the substance to which he is allergic. This stimulates production of the appropriate blocking antibodies so that, if the individual encounters a full-scale exposure, his alerted immune system will be able to neutralize the antigen. Actually the best way to eliminate an allergy to dust or pollen or mold would be to avoid it completely, but our lifestyles are far too complex for that. To date, no conventional system of inoculation has been developed for food allergies, and it may indeed be a fact that food allergies involve a different mechanism from other allergic conditions. Some researchers have suggested, for example, that food allergy or intolerance results from a deficiency or malfunction of the digestive enzymes. Because of this, we aren't even sure that antibody stimulation would be effective with this type of problem. The clinical ecologists, however, believe they have found a successful alternative to the desensitization process of inoculation: exposing the individual to minute but gradually increasing amounts of extracts of the foods to which he is sensitive until an acceptable tolerance level is established.

As with any medical condition in which claims are made on the basis of clinical evidence rather than classical research studies, the subject of food allergy is capable of eliciting strong opinions on both sides. Clinicians who have watched patients improve, after identifying troublesome foods and establishing a diet to avoid the troublemakers, can become impatient with others who discuss the need for controlled studies to verify the scientific and clinical validity of the concept.

Theoretical discussions aside, food allergies were fundamentally implicated in a new condition medicine identified in the early fifties—hyperactivity in children. Although not recognized as a problem until mid-century, hyperactivity has now become almost a household word. A hyperactive child is often characterized as "having behavior problems," meaning that he appears spoiled, self-centered, and unresponsive to discipline. Such children are frequently "on" one minute and depressed and irritable the next. Because of their mood swings, they often require constant attention and discipline. Although initially thought to be an isolated phenomenon, hyperactivity is now known to occur fairly regularly in our population. Conventional treatment requires the use of drugs to calm the child so that he can control his actions and direct himself toward more constructive behavior.

Generally considered a behavioral problem, with symptom management as its fundamental treatment, childhood hyperactivity was left to the backwaters of medicine reserved for conditions we don't really understand and tend to feel frustrated about. Somewhere along the line it must have appeared odd to someone that this condition was almost nonexistent until the middle of the twentieth century. Coincidentally it was at mid-century that our food supply underwent substantial change, specifically an increase in processed food and the use of food additives such as preservatives, artificial flavors, and food dyes. Much of this was done in an attempt to make food last longer, to make it more convenient for the growing number of middle-American housewives, and to add to its visual and taste appeal. If you were to review the records the federal government uses to track such things, you might be surprised to learn that between the late fifties and mid-seventies the amount of substances added to our food has more than doubled. Right now, on average, each of us consumes almost five pounds of food additives annually.[4] Presumably if you have a problem with your digestive system related to the chemical composition of food, the addition of such a variety of substances would have a significant effect on your health and well-being.

Currently the government estimates that the number of additives used in our food falls somewhere between 3,000 and 10,000.[5] For hyperactive children and their families the practical advantages of using such additive-laden products has been far overridden by the discovery that many children are highly sensitive to these substances, some to the point of absolute intolerance.[6] In many of these children the ingestion of specific kinds of food additives can cause the short-circuit that results in their abnormal behavior. The literature on pediatric hyperactivity is full of inspiring case histories in which symptom relief became almost immediate when the child was restricted to unprocessed, natural foods. For some children, however, understanding their sensitivity to synthetic foods and additives proved only the first step. Although removal of chemical allergens from the diet usually produced a substantial effect, sometimes it was not enough.

So, working with the success of an additive-free diet, scientists and clinicians proceeded to examine other possible allergens in the environment to which a child might be reactive. After substantial clinical investigation, it was established that children still experiencing difficulty after synthetics and additives were removed from their diet could be helped by elimination of particular irritating foods. Again, the literature is replete with case studies of unhappy and unproductive children who were found to be sensitive to any of a wide range of foods, from dairy products to vegetables. Generally, once the child's allergy was identified and an appropriate replacement diet designed, he was able to go on to lead a more normal life.[7]

Other documented but less common effects of food sensitivity include criminal behavior in adolescents and young adults. One explanation suggests that the tissue swelling that often results from an allergic reaction can intefere with the normal function of the brain, which in turn exhibits itself as abnormal or antisocial behavior. The limited research completed thus far indicates that such individuals could be rehabilitated if they were to eliminate the offending antigens from their environment.[8] Researchers have also explored the possible relationship between food allergies and mental illness in adults. Cause-and-effect links have been established between the ingestion of certain foods and subsequent exacerbations of mental illnesses such as schizophrenia.[9] Whether this is an allergic reaction to food, a sensitivity to food additives, or some kind of chemical imbalance caused by inadequate nutrition has not yet been conclusively established.

Although these and other speculations await more research, ample clinical evidence has established that, for food-sensitive individuals, there is indeed a connection between ingestion of foods to which they are individually susceptible and the subsequent manifestation of discomfort and illness. Well-conducted studies have verified the impressions of literally tens of thousands of people that certain foods can make them acutely ill.[10]

One of the most common problems resulting from food intolerance is abdominal colic. Generally, colic refers to the body's inability to absorb a particular food. Most of us think of it in relation to an infant's difficulty in digesting milk. In reality colic can be a bother at any age. The very uncomfortable bloated feeling it produces results from the body's attempt to rid itself of something it can't digest. Unfortunately, the irritating substance moves through the intestines at the same rate as food the body can tolerate and is subjected to the same digestive processes. The typical symptoms of allergy-induced colic begin to appear about an hour after eating, as the food leaves the stomach and starts to enter the intestines, although the reaction may take as long as eight hours to manifest itself. The gas usually associated with this unpleasant condition extends the abdomen and increases the discomfort. This gas results from increased bacterial growth from the undigested food. The longer the irritating food remains in the system, the greater the discomfort. When the body finally succeeds in eliminating the offending material the result is usually diarrhea until the system is completely cleared out.

At one time or another we have all had occasion to listen to a friend tell the story of how his breathing was impaired for hours after he ate a small piece of avocado; how his eyes puffed up after he inadvertently wolfed down a handful of pecans; how, on an occasion of eating shellfish, his mother was horrified to discover red blotches on her face and hands. If the reaction happens more than once, and if your friend is a reasonably bright person, he has probably figured out that such foods should be avoided. People who experience this kind of reaction may be luckier than those who suffer with symptoms in the digestive tract, because the former provides very explicit and undeniable proof of a food reaction, whereas the latter can linger as chronic, undiagnosed illness.

The mechanism responsible for common allergic reactions is the antibody immunoglobulin E (IgE). The combination of these antibodies with specific allergens and (mast) tissue cells triggers the release of chemicals that constrict the blood vessels in the tissues. The result is edema (or swelling), usually occurring around the face but which may be evident anywhere in the body. This type of dramatic reaction establishes a graphically definitive link between eating an irritating food and the corresponding allergic reaction. Unless your storyteller has an usually high tolerance for discomfort and pain, he or she will undoubtedly strive to avoid that food in the future.

In addition to this inflamed tissue response, problems in the respiratory tract are a common reaction to allergy.

Uttering the words *food allergy* in a group of people usually produces a story about a respiratory attack that followed a meal of shellfish, or meat, or vegetables, or whatever. Such attacks do occur, in similar fashion to hives and other skin reactions, and they are often more dramatic than gastrointestinal symptoms because they can be mysterious and dangerous. Asthmatic attacks, for example, have been known to occur up to two days after eating a food to which the individual is sensitive. Frequently a food-induced asthma attack may be accompanied by other symptoms, especially in children and young adults. Thus, it would not be unusual to see a young child manifesting secondary asthmatic symptoms of chronic irritability, insomnia, abdominal pain, and skin rashes. In adults the reaction may be equally intense: depression, joint pain similar to that from arthritis, increased frequency of urination, and fatigue.

Orlanda Brown, now an adult, survived the usual diseases of childhood—mumps, chicken pox, the measles—without much thought, along with the usual quota of colds, earaches, and sore throats. Looking back, she says she can remember an occasional stomachache now and then, although neither she nor her parents took much notice.

Orlanda's childhood was characterized by its regularity. She comes from a middle-class Connecticut family. Her mother's ancestors descended from the original colonists, and her father considers himself a regular Connecticut Yankee. Like her brother and older sister, Orlanda went to the local public schools. She planned to be a nurse and selected a small liberal arts college in northern Vermont.

It was during her first year of college that Orlanda's difficulties surfaced. Settled comfortably in a turn-of-the-century dormitory, with a roommate from Brewster, a small town on Cape Cod, Orlanda busied herself with getting to know the college, understanding the written and unwritten rules of university life, and deciding that she liked the school and her major. She was well into her first semester when she noticed she hadn't been feeling well. At first she thought it was the dorm food, so her initial response was to stick with her usual foods and not eat anything exotic. Caught up in the excitement of her first semester at college, she chalked it all up to nerves. In the back of her mind she remembered the stomachaches from her childhood but didn't put two and two together until she began to experience dizzy spells.

She describes it:

"A day would be going along OK; I would be walking across campus or sitting at my desk doing homework, feeling pretty good about myself and what I was doing. Then just like that, I'd start to feel faint and disoriented. Sometimes I actually forgot where I was. I started to get a little frightened."

She told her mother about it one evening on the phone, and they agreed that she should get more sleep. Orlanda promised she'd watch herself carefully for a couple of weeks, and her mother suggested that if she didn't start feeling better soon, she should see a doctor. Orlanda decided to keep a daily record of how she felt, recording entries before breakfast, at lunch, at dinner, and before she got into bed at night. She was amazed to find a list of recurrent and related symptoms. Her stomachaches were occurring almost every day and were followed by bloating and diarrhea. She also noticed that her dizzy spells often preceded a severe headache and a sore throat. She went home for Thanksgiving expecting that a week of her mother's cooking and her own bed would probably straighten her out. She didn't want to alarm her family, and she wasn't particularly interested in going to the doctor to find out there was something really wrong—and then perhaps missing school.

Although she began to feel a little better at home, back at school she grew worse. The nausea began to bother her so much that all she could eat was whole-wheat rolls. She stayed in her room, while her roommate went down to dinner, and waited for the roll and butter she would bring back for her. Home for Christmas, Orlanda was uncomfortable and obviously underweight, and her alarmed parents insisted she see a doctor.

She remembers her symptoms:

"I was just lying around all the time, and that wasn't like me. I had worked as a volunteer in the hospital while I was in

high school, and I figured I'd do that again over vacation. It was an opportunity for an experience that I really enjoyed. But I was so sick then that I couldn't do anything. I'd just get up in the morning, eat a little something—some whole-wheat crackers and a grapefruit usually—and then the headaches would start and I'd have to lie down on the couch or go back to bed. Sometimes I wouldn't feel too bad in the morning. I might even wake up feeling like I had a good night's sleep. But by dinnertime I was feeling so bad that I couldn't even eat with the family. So they made me go to the hospital.

"At the hospital they ran all sorts of tests. It seemed obvious to everyone that something was wrong. I couldn't eat; I was losing weight. They kept giving me more and more sophisticated tests, even a spinal tap. But they couldn't find out what was wrong with me. Every day one of the doctors would come in and ask me how I felt, which I thought was pretty obvious. I got to the point that I just wanted them to go away. My mother's friends felt sorry for me—being in the hospital during Christmastime—but they only made it worse. They'd come in and say things like, 'There, there, dear, we know it's just the strain of going to school and all of that. You just stay here and get a good rest, and you'll be better in no time.' Or they'd question me: 'Maybe you're just worried about something and you don't realize it.'

"Now, when you're sick and the doctors know what's wrong with you, your friends know how to act. They can say, 'Yeah, I had that or I know someone who had that and you'll be OK in a week.' But when you're in the hospital feeling awful, taking up a bed and costing lots of money, and they can't figure out what the problem is, then people end up looking at you like you're weird. They don't know what to say because they don't know what you've got. They can't bring you chicken soup because that's for colds and you don't have a cold, even though you have a headache and a sore throat. And hot tea is for stomach flu, but you don't have that 'cause you can eat some things. They just don't know how to act. And so what usually happens is they fall back on something lame like 'There must be something bothering her. She's not adjusting well, or maybe her parents are having problems, or

*maybe she really hates college and doesn't want to tell them.'
They get impatient with you. They begin to suspect that
maybe you don't want to get better."*

So Orlanda went home with a prescription for extra-
strength Tylenol and a lot of anger. Her parents were baffled
and concerned. She'd never been that sick before nor for so
long.

*"We thought about allergies, but it was the conventional
stuff. My mom thought it was the laundry soap and went nuts
changing brands, but that couldn't have been it because I was
also sick at school. Then she thought about the material in
the sheets and the type of cleaner she used in the house. We
also considered that I might be allergic to cigarette smoke
because both of my parents smoke, but I didn't think so
because my roommate at college didn't smoke, and I was even
sicker while I was at school. They were constantly asking me
questions: 'How do you feel? How's your head?' I got to the
point where I didn't want to answer anymore; it was very
frustrating. The worst time was when I was in the hospital,
because sometimes I got so bad I couldn't talk.*

*"While I was there in the hospital and all those people were
saying maybe I was having problems that I was trying to
cover up, I called my sister, who's a nurse, and I said to her,
'Maybe I'm doing this to myself.' She told me not to be silly
and that they'd find out what was wrong with me. I tried to
believe her, but I hurt from all those needles they'd stuck me
with, and I looked terrible from all the weight I'd lost. I felt so
weak that after I got home I couldn't even get up off the
couch. When I did get up I had trouble sitting up straight, and
I walked funny."*

A friend of Orlanda's family finally suggested she see an
allergist, which she did. When he tested her, however, she
didn't show any of the conventional allergies. She asked him
about food allergies, and he told her that he knew about a
physician who was working in that area but that he wasn't
very sure about what he was doing. Orlanda took the
number and called. Her new doctor recognized that something was wrong and took the time to talk to her about it. She
turned out to be allergic to wheat, milk, citrus fruit, and red

meat. When she told him she was existing on grapefruit and crackers he immediately suspected both foods. Orlanda fasted for five days to clean out her system and then gradually began to add back foods one at a time. She found she could tolerate chicken and cooked green beans, canned tuna, and salmon. She stayed with those foods for a while and then gradually added some others. Some she tolerated; others she didn't.

"I'm still trying to find out if there are other things that bother me because I'm still not completely all right. My stomach gets upset sometimes, but my dizzy spells and headaches are gone. We think it might be an additive or something like that. But compared to staying in bed and moaning, I'm OK. I went back to my volunteer job at the hospital because I lost so much time I couldn't attend college in the spring semester. I ran into one of my doctors at work, and he asked me how I felt. I jabbered at him about what I was doing, and I suppose it did sound a little strange. He probably thought I was neurotic, but that's OK because he probably thought that when I was in the hospital. He finally just gave me a pat on the shoulder and said that if I was feeling better, I'd better stick to what I was doing. But I know he thought I was just a bundle of nerves."

Orlanda exhibited a wide range of symptoms, partly because she did an excellent job of eating the specific foods that irritated her. Whenever she didn't feel like eating, she chose the very foods that made her sick. Although to her they seemed like the only things she could tolerate, she would have been better had she eaten nothing at all.

The type of headache Orlanda suffered from is a frequent result of food allergies. Often characterized as a tension headache, it usually involves a dull, nagging pain in the back of the head and neck and sometimes the temples. Although similar symptoms can result from stress or overwork, a daily headache, especially over a substantial period of time such as Orlanda had, is often indicative of food allergy. Migraine headaches have also been associated with allergic reactions to food.[11] The symptoms of migraine are similar to what Orlanda suffered when she had a dizzy spell followed by an intense headache. Migraines are also frequently associated with temporary loss of sight or blurred vision, or they can cause numbness, weakness, and loss of balance.

Those individuals who frequently experience migraine attacks have been found to experience a variety of chemical changes in their blood, specifically the presence of several powerful vasoconstrictors, which can cause the blood vessels to contract or become spastic. That food allergies are related to migraine headaches has been suspected for more than a century; in fact, the clinical descriptions that implicated food allergies as an underlying cause of migraine headaches were noted as early as 1873.[12]

Orlanda's case not only demonstrates the wide range of symptoms that can result from food allergies, it also illustrates a fundamental characteristic of the condition—it is often the foods that we most frequently eat, like, and consider "safe" which turn out to be our allergens.

An initial step to be applied if you are interested in determining your possible allergies is to consider the following six questions.

1. Do you think you might be allergic to a food or foods? If so, which one(s)?
2. Are you aware of any foods that you eat at least two or three times a week which you're sure you're not allergic to?
3. What are your favorite foods?
4. Are there any foods that you consume at least once every day or two? What are they?
5. What foods do you presently eat that you think you could give up most easily if you found you were allergic to them?
6. What foods would cause you the most hardship if you had to give them up?[13]

You may have guessed that these questions are "loaded." The work of researchers in correlating symptom relief with food intake has produced some basic facts about the behavior of food allergies. First, the foods we like the most and consume most often are the ones to which we are most likely to be allergic. Second, those foods we don't particularly care about are probably our safe foods. One rule of thumb is that, if you have a feeling of satisfaction and contentment after eating a particular food, the odds are you're allergic to it. In other words, if you crave it, you should watch out for it.

Interestingly enough, if an individual who is allergic to a certain food avoids that food for a few days, he will probably experience withdrawal symptoms and feel terrible. If he continues to avoid the food for a few more days, the symptoms will go away. In fact, one difficulty in diagnosing food allergies is that regular consumption of an offending food "masks" the allergic reaction. The body is able to cover up an allergy for years without a hint of its underlying effects. Eventually, however, the body will lose its capacity to tolerate the constant irritation, and the symptoms of food allergy will erupt. Orlanda, for example, was able to eat wheat throughout most of her childhood. Finally, as a young adult, she manifested the result of the cumulative allergic effect. It is possible that the stress of going away to school could have precipitated the eruption of her allergy. It is probably more likely, however, that under the pressure of her first year in college, she fell back on eating the foods she liked most because they gave her a sense of well-being. This in turn produced an overload on an already overworked system. So, aside from the discomfort and pain of a chronic headache or the unsightliness of a puffy face, the constant irritation of an unacknowledged food allergy can lead from chronic indigestion to colitis, and further expose the individual to the risk of all colitis sufferers, intestinal cancer.

This masking of an allergy—by frequent addictive use of a food—is responsible for the popular misconception that you can "outgrow" an allergy. In reality an allergy never disappears; it just goes underground. Things appear to be quiet during what is referred to as the *accommodation stage,* but it is only a matter of time before the body signals its inability to continue its tolerance of the irritation. The fact that abstaining from an allergic food for a few days produces withdrawal symptoms provides a clear indication of an allergy's effect on the body.

One food allergy specialist believes that consuming food to which you're allergic can result in effects as deteriorating to the body's metabolism as the addictive use of alcohol or narcotics. This view considers allergy, food or otherwise, not a trivial disturbance peculiar to one individual or another, but a major systemic condition that should be controlled.[14]

So, even of itself, food allergy is not an illness to be taken lightly. Combined with the malfunction in the immunological system, which can expose an individual to the risk of multiple sclerosis, it becomes a formidable challenge indeed.

6

OTHER
RESEARCH RESULTS

There is comfort in certainty.

Having knowledge, of course, is one way to be certain. On the other hand, lack of knowledge can be disturbing and anxiety-producing. Our understanding of multiple sclerosis is shaky because our theories continue to evolve. And although vitality is one enticing aspect of theory-in-the-making, achieving "the answer" to a perplexing question is far more reinforcing. After so much hide-and-seek, it can indeed be comfortable to "know."

Multiple sclerosis continues to provide researchers with a vital and complex challenge. On some days it appears that the more we discover, the more complicated the problem becomes. The science of immunology, however, has matured markedly, especially over the last twenty years, encouraged partially by technological advances which have made it possible to isolate and study parts of the human body never before available. Indeed, our scrutiny of the immune system has identified a number of productive avenues in our investigation of the disease that is multiple sclerosis.

The facts about MS fall into several categories. Although

recent work continues to suggest the importance of a virus, we are nonetheless expanding our appreciation of how the immune system contributes to the onset and continued clinical course of the disease. As is generally the case, the known has spawned speculation and thus encouraged further investigation. After all, without a reasonable hunch to pursue, even the best scientist is at a standstill. We present here as much as is certain about the etiology and cause of MS, some of which has provided the basis for the theory that is the cornerstone of this book. Additionally, we have allowed ourselves the luxury of engaging in a few hunches and speculations of our own, based on current work.

Multiple sclerosis is classified as a demyelinating disease, which means that it manifests itself as patchy areas of inflammation and demyelination in the white matter of the brain and spinal cord. As we have seen, this primary demyelination, as it is called, results in the breakdown of the myelin or insulation covering the nerve fibers in the central nervous system (CNS). Destruction is selective, in that the nerve cells (neurons) with their long fibers (axons) for the most part remain intact. However, the cells composing the myelin, the oligodendrocytes, are lost. Demyelination slows down the conduction of signals within the nervous system, which can in turn cause loss of coordination, often paralysis, and sometimes death.

Despite considerable research efforts, we still don't know how this demyelination occurs. As we have indicated, two hypotheses have emerged and provided the framework for current research. One of these hypotheses, which at first simply implicated a virus as the cause of MS, has been peered and poked at from a variety of angles, with the result that its original, simple thought has been expanded. We now consider that although a virus doesn't "cause" the disease— as a virus might cause the flu—its presence may interfere with the normal function of the immune system. This thought has in turn generated speculation that some individuals may have a genetic defect predisposing them to a particular virus or viruses or inhibiting their ability to react appropriately to a viral infection. The most obvious conclusion resulting from this cross-fertilization between the viral and autoimmune studies is that the "answer" may be far more complex than originally thought and will undoubtedly require considerable additional work before we're finished.

A number of clinical observations have led investigators to attempt to isolate a specific virus as the cause of MS. We have already mentioned that MS is more prevalent in northern, as opposed to southern, climates, specifically northern Europe and North America. There is the additional fact that individuals who move from the south to the north before the age of fifteen have an increased risk of contracting the disease like those born in the north. Persons moving south before age fifteen, on the other hand, enjoy a similar decreased risk as others in the more southern climates. Such observations, as potentially fruitful as they once seemed, have basically been played out. To date, all attempts to isolate a specific virus in tissue from MS patients or by inoculation in primates have failed, as have more sophisticated laboratory experiments in cross-cultivation.[1]

As we have noted, however, viruses have not been completely cleared of a substantive role in the disease. Concurrent with the work to isolate an MS-specific virus, immunologists have continued to investigate a possible malfunction in the immune system that might contribute to the development of multiple sclerosis. Happily, their efforts have identified three productive areas of investigation. The first involves potential inadequacies in humoral immunity, particularly the release of antibodies. The suggestion is that there may be a virus capable of confusing the immune system so that appropriate antibodies aren't activated, which allows the virus the time it needs to "settle in." A second suggestion relates to potential problems with cell-mediated immunity. The two possibilities which continue to be investigated are that an individual's white blood cells don't react properly against a specific virus or that they exhibit an inadequate degree of reaction. In either case the effect is the same: the virus spreads without restriction. The third area of research involves a possible overreaction by the attacking white blood cells, perhaps because of a lack of suppressor cells.

The first important step forward in the investigation of MS was the capability of duplicating a model to study the disease. Scientifically, a model serves the important function of demonstrating how a disease "works" and hopefully produces clues as to how to control it. In the case of multiple sclerosis scientists have been able to produce a relapsing disease called *experimental allergic encephalomyelitis* (EAE) in laboratory animals. To do so, the subjects are inoculated with nervous-system tissue. Using standard laboratory procedures, the injected material is enhanced with killed tuberculosis organisms, which increases the likelihood that the animal's immune system will become sensitized. In most instances the animal will exhibit a disease in which the symptoms are not unlike multiple sclerosis in many respects. Such work has documented a now recognized fact essential to the Autoimmune Theory for MS—that a component of myelin in the nervous system is not recognized as self by the mature immune system. Therefore, this myelin substance is capable of evoking a foreign body response.

As research techniques have became more refined, however, it has become possible to produce a more purified form of myelin for EAE inoculation, called *basic myelin protein* (BP). Interestingly enough, this new, purified substance produces different symptoms from the initially used, cruder material. Although the resulting disease is similar, its course has less resemblance to MS.[2] An obvious interpetation of these findings is that the mechanism that initiates MS may involve a sensitization to more than the basic myelin protein in the central nervous system. It could even be that one of the other components of the cruder myelin preparation is actually the antigenic substance rather than, as we have previously thought, the myelin itself.

Such findings seem to suggest both that the precipitating cause for MS is more than a simple sensitivity to myelin and that subsequent attacks might result from a more complicated reaction of the immune system than scientists first envisioned. Either the presence of another kind of substance is needed, such as an additional component of the nerve sheath, or the inclusion of another mechanism, which unpredictably malfunctions, is needed. Further, this thought supports the oft-voiced contention that the allergic reaction to myelin is of such low magnitude that by itself it will not cause an attack of MS.

There is the additional consideration that, in laboratory tests with EAE, the sensitizing substance is injected directly into the body of the lab animal. This action initiates the reaction of the animal's peripheral immune system. Thus, not only is the animal sensitized to the myelin of the inoculation, but a generalized sensitization occurs against the myelin in its own nervous system, producing the symptoms of EAE. As we have noted, the blood-brain barrier in humans normally prevents direct sensitization of the white blood cells to the central nervous system. These results support the necessity of identifying the element that causes our white blood cells to be introduced to the CNS antigen, as well as whatever factor makes it possible for that introduction to happen. If some mechanism didn't exist whereby the immune system could react to the antigenic substance in the CNS, we would have no MS.

The exact nature of the immune response associated with whatever viruses may be implicated in MS has also become the subject of much interest and research. Studies have dealt particularly with the possible cause for persistence of viruses in tissues, so as to account for the fact that such viruses tend to escape detection and subsequent destruction by the immune system. An additional question, which still does not have a plausible answer, is why, after a latent period, such a virus should initiate renewed inflammation. It was originally thought that a fault in cell-mediated immunity, possibly inherited, might exist. Other alternatives have included speculation that the long-term existence of a virus in a cell may alter the antigenic character of the cell itself. This could then mean that the host cells themselves might evoke a foreign-body response.

Taking such clues as the basis for possible research hypotheses, much early work in this area centered on a search for antibodies directed generally against the nervous system, particularly myelin. Typically in this kind of research, an important step would be to attempt to relate specific antibodies to specific viruses because where there are antibodies there also must be a virus. Attempts to find a virus to account for most of the excess antibodies, however, were universally unsuccessful, adding another blow to a simple viral etiology. However, the examination of the blood of MS patients necessary to conduct such tests revealed a number of substantial differences between the blood of MS-afflicted individuals and normal subjects. One research study, for example, did report higher levels of antibodies to measles virus in the sera (the liquid part of the blood) in MS patients.[3] The same rearchers also reported that more MS patients than individuals in the control group had antibodies to measles, rubella, and vaccinia viruses in their spinal fluid.[4] Because it has by now become fairly obvious that a virus doesn't "cause" MS per se, but is somehow implicated, such findings have supported speculation that a virus somehow may activate the immune system of MS patients, perhaps fallaciously, and initiate the chain of events whereby the individual becomes sensitized to myelin.

Another interesting finding concerns the identification of specific factors in the blood of MS patients. A factor is an agent or element, such as a chemical compound, that contributes to the production of a specific effect. With the advent of new techniques for culturing central nervous system tissue in the laboratory, factors have been found in the sera of MS patients which cause demyelination and block nerve conduction.[5] Indeed, it is a fact that as early as 1961 researchers reported demyelinating factors in the sera of laboratory animals with EAE, as well as in the sera of patients with MS.[6] Although originally some of these factors appeared to be similar to antibodies, current work suggests that they may be enzymes that are released by the white blood cells. Regardless of their origin, their presence could mean that the MS-afflicted individual actually produces, within his own system, those chemicals that cause the demyelination of the nerve covering. As in all things having to do with the CNS, this is a complicated business, requiring the presence of a number of other elements or chemicals to produce the resulting effect. Again we go back to the suggestion that a virus might stimulate the production of such chemicals or that the reaction might result from a problem in the immune system with which the individual was born.

In this regard it is important to consider recent developments in MS diagnosis. Particularly significant among the laboratory tests used to confirm the occurrence of MS are those which detect the presence of antibodies in spinal fluid. For many years, it was possible to elicit an elevated gamma globulin level in the spinal fluid of MS patients. This routinely occurred in approximately 60–70 percent of the cases. Since most antibodies are gamma globulins, such findings indicate a high level of antibodies and intense immune system surveillance. New techniques have recently been developed which separate these gamma globulins, or antibodies, as they are found in the spinal fluid into fractions called *oligoclonal* or *monoclonal bands*. This, in turn, has made it possible to pinpoint even more precisely which of the globulins are in fact antibodies.[7] With the advent of this method for evaluating spinal fluid, up to 95 percent of MS patients have demonstrated abnormal results, although this test is still not capable of yielding a specific diagnosis of MS. Additionally, a similar pattern of oligoclonal banding of antibodies has also been found in the MS plaques themselves as they exist in the central nervous system.[8] Such results would seem to confirm that MS patients are reacting in a different immunological fashion than normal subjects.

As we pursue investigation of the exact type of anomaly in the immune system that might contribute to MS, we necessarily encounter another interesting aspect of MS research—interferon. Interferon is a type of protein produced by the cells of the body during a viral infection. In addition to its function of protecting cells from infection, interferon has wide-ranging general effects on the activities of the immune system. To understand the potential role played by interferon in MS, we must refer back to our discussion of the various types and functions of white blood cells. You will remember that a certain kind of T-cell, the Killer Ts or K-cells, is responsible for attacks on contaminated cells, whether they contain a virus, a tumor, or are cells from a transplanted organ. These K-cells are antigen-specific in that they are tagged for specific kinds of cells with which to react. The T-cells are antigen-specific in that they are tagged for specific whole-cell reactions, and these antibodies interact with the target cells. B-cells, on the other hand, produce antibodies to specific antigens. B-cells appear to originate and remain around the bowel, where one of their activities is to make it easier for cells in that area to gobble up waste products. The B-cells also evolve into plasma cells, which turn out to be the most powerful antibody-producing cells. Thus B-cells and their successors, the plasma cells, exert their influence in humoral immunity, in contrast to the cell-mediated immunity of the T-cells.

Although powerful, the Bs don't work completely in isolation. Significantly, the T-cells do influence the B-cells' function. They do this through appropriate enhancement or repression of B-cell activity. It has not been determined definitively, but it has been suggested that the active T-cells—the Killer Ts or K-cells—actually form a third general group of white blood cells called *Null cells*. Null cells are so named because they lack the morphological characteristics that identify the B- and T-cells. Regardless of their facelessness, the Null cells are extremely important because they also may function as cytotoxic or killer cells. Some are called NK-cells, for natural killer cells, because, unlike the Bs and Ts, they do not require antibody for their function.

It has been established that interferon appears to enhance the cytotoxic activity of the NK-cells.[9] Thus, the question has arisen whether a lack of this substance may predispose an individual to viral infection or may prevent adequate elimination of such an infection. In other words, if some form of genetic defect caused a deficiency in the production of interferon, the entire function of an individual's attack cells could be thrown off. Interestingly, one study has indicated that approximately 30 percent of MS patients examined showed a decreased ability to produce interferon, and that NK cell activity was reduced in about 30 percent of the cases.[10] Both of these findings could mean that an individual conceivably could be left unequipped to effectively combat the presence of a dangerous virus. Likewise, several other investigators have found evidence of reduced function in the NK-cell population of MS patients.[11] Although one explanation for reduced activity of the NK-cells could be a decreased output of interferon, it has also been shown that, even with added interferon, the NK-cells in such individuals responded less well than normal controls.[12] Aside from some malfunction in their production of interferon, this would also seem to indicate defective function in the NK-cells themselves.

In any case, although we are not actually sure about what is happening in such circumstances, we are close enough to some interesting findings to allow ourselves some speculation. If, for example, an individual had some genetic defect in his Killer T-cells or in the production of those chemicals which initiate their work, the chances are increased that those cells would be inadequate in number and intensity to seek out and neutralize an invading virus or other antigenic substance. This would explain why the virus has a chance to obtain a foothold in the body, allowing it traveling time into the central nervous system.

Interesting as these thoughts might be, results from other areas indicate there may be a problem with the mechanism of the suppressor T-cells in closing down an attack after a foreign threat has been mastered. Such information emerges from research on prostaglandins. As with interferon, the study of prostaglandins is a relatively new but extremely exciting field, not only regarding MS but other diseases and conditions as well. Prostaglandins are released from white blood cells when the cell membranes become disrupted or broken down. A major source of prostaglandins, therefore, is the intestinal tract because of the large number of white blood cells lining the bowel wall. Disruption of white blood cell membranes occurs when the cells come in contact with substances to which they're sensitized. As we have seen, this can be any antigenic substance, including a virus, or food, or endotoxin. Significant to our discussion of possible reduced function of the attack white blood cells, one researcher has discovered that prostaglandins inhibit NK-cell function.[13] This finding is especially interesting in view of the fact that other researchers have reported reduced NK-cell activity among MS patients. [14] Supporting this thought, one group of investigators has also shown that monocytes from MS patients "spontaneously" secrete increased levels of prostaglandins.[15]

Let's consider how these findings may be interrelated. First, remember that much of the prostaglandins are released from white blood cells in the intestines. Second, the white blood cells release this material only if they experience a breakdown of their cell membranes, which usually happens if they come in contact with an antigenic substance. Aside from a virus, the two types of common antigens existing in the bowel area are irritating foods the body is attempting to digest and endotoxin released from bacteria as part of this process.

In terms of our theory, this means that someone who is eating a food to which he is allergic would be increasing the production of prostaglandins in his body, either through the direct action of the irritating food or as a result of the endotoxin produced as the food is digested. These prostaglandins then inhibit the action of the natural Killer (NK) cells, which can function to keep a latent or persistent viral infection in check. Added to this is the possibility that an individual may have a problem with his suppressor cells. Inadequate suppression of immune activity may permit unrestrained attack by one's own white blood cells on the myelin. Stopping the production of prostaglandins—by controlling the infection or abstinence from the irritating food—might relax the whole process and allow the suppressor cells a chance to do their work.

Confirmation of this thought comes from a clinical study involving colitis and food allergies. It is a well-known clinical fact that aspirin inhibits the release of prostaglandins. Based on this consideration, a study was designed in which a group of individuals with food allergies took aspirin before they attempted to eat the foods to which they are allergic. The aspirin made it possible to control the release of prostaglandins, which enabled the subjects to eat their troublesome food without the usual uncomfortable reactions. The same procedure was attempted with another group of subjects diagnosed as suffering from ulcerative colitis. Those participating were encouraged to identify the foods that bothered them as possible allergies (by virtue of observable clinical symptoms) and to avoid them. Avoidance of the irritating foods confirmed the food allergies. The foods were subsequently reintroduced, coupled with the use of aspirin before eating. As with the first group, the appearance of symptoms, formerly diagnosed as colitis, was diminished.[16]

Further research concerning immune regulation by white blood cells, particularly T-cells, should prove extremely valuable. At the present time this area appears to be one of the most promising for our understanding of MS. One recent result of this work, for example, has been the development of specific monoclonal antibodies against different types of immunoregulatory T-cell subsets.[17] One study has noted that patients with reduced numbers of suppressor cells from T8 subset may have a more severe course of MS. This suggests that we might develop particular therapies based on types of T-cell abnormalities which can exist and then select corresponding patients for treatment.

Very exciting information finally has come also from a report describing recurring attacks of confusion and unsteadiness occuring in patients who have undergone a small-bowel shunting procedure, jejunoileostomy, for obesity.[18] [19] It appears that this procedure may result in undigested carbohydrates reaching the lower bowel where bacteria then may act on this food and produce a sugar from glucose, d-lactate, that cannot be metabolized. Since the nervous system is dependent upon proper glucose metabolism for energy and nutrition, nerve cell malfunction and cell death may result from this. One might speculate that a food allergy also may create a similar situation by causing the rapid shunting of undigested food through the small bowel. As a result of excessive production of d-lactate, aggravated symptoms of latent multiple sclerosis might appear. Certainly this is an aspect of this complicated disease that should be investigated thoroughly.

A hypothesis is a hunch, an informed guess, an inspiration, the product of an inquisitive mind. It is necessary, but only the beginning. Without a hypothesis we would have to forget definitive research. What must follow the hypothesis, of course, is a well-designed and well-executed research project. Nothing definitive ever comes of a sloppy study. In relation to MS, we are still being guided by more hunches than actual facts. Our expertise in studying the nervous system, however, and more importantly the immune system, has grown considerably in recent years. We have more opportunities than ever before, as well as more challenges. That much is certain.

In effect, the simple viral hypothesis for MS has reached its deadend. When one possible research track dries up, the result is often renewed enthusiasm and vigor for its alternatives—in this case, an autoimmune explanation for the disease. Out of this work has come an increased appreciation of how the immune system protects the body from invaders. Specifically, we have achieved a more comprehensive understanding of the action of our white blood cells, a fascinating story in itself.

In the early days of live television broadcasters had a quick response when things went wrong with the picture and they had exhausted all their resources. The screen would blacken for a few seconds, and then a printed card would appear, asking for the viewers' goodwill. It's the nature of medical research that the answer to a perplexing problem can be found in one study or hide for years from its pursuers. We don't know all the answers pertaining to MS yet, but we're close. So your best strategy may be to recall the patience needed in those early TV years, and *Stay Tuned*.

Unlike those first TV viewers, however, there are things you can do about your MS, here and now, that can make your wait for the definitive answer much easier.

7

DETECTING YOUR FOOD ALLERGIES

Jonathan is ten years old. He is just about average for his age: not too tall, or short, or round. He wears glasses, or is supposed to. Most of the time they're at the bottom of his pack, along with the toad. Jonathan has sandy-colored hair and shoelaces that are never tied. His shoes are probably the least of his problems, however, because Jonathan is what is called *learning disabled,* which means he doesn't assimilate information as quickly as normal children and he has difficulty learning basic skills. Jonathan also has difficulty paying attention in class. Until about six months ago he usually distinguished himself by routinely not doing what he was asked to do. But about that time a new lady appeared at school. They called her a *nutritionist.* She talked to Jonathan about what he ate. She seemed to be very concerned about the colas and the fruit sticks and the cheese sandwiches. The oranges seemed to bother her a lot, too—he was eating about eight oranges a day back then. She told him he ought to stop eating so many oranges. She even suggested that perhaps he should stop eating oranges altogether. When he didn't respond to her suggestion, the nutritionist explained to Jonathan that oranges, at least as many as he was eating, weren't good for him.

Jonathan didn't really care that much about oranges. He ate them because his mother packed them for his lunch. He could also eat them during break at school, and there were always some around when he got home at night. So when the nutritionist asked him to stop eating oranges for a while and pick another fruit, he didn't really care. First, though, he had to go a week without any fruit at all. He thought he could do that. To everyone's surprise, including his own, Jonathan's behavior changed. He sat in class and did what he was told. Everyone seemed to be happy with him, and he didn't mind it himself.

After two weeks they told him he could eat any other fruits he thought he might like. He chose bananas and pears. In fact, he decided he liked the bananas so much that pretty soon he was eating eight, ten bananas a day. He liked them because they weren't as messy as oranges. This went on for a while, and then things started getting bad again. He couldn't sit still in class, and the teachers were on his back. Finally he went back to see the nutritionist. She told him the bananas weren't working and she thought they would have to figure out a better system for Jonathan's snacks. From now on he could eat a lot of different fruits instead of the same one every day. He could have the same fruit twice a week, but no more. He did what he was told—the fruit didn't really matter to him anyhow—and things got better again.

It is generally considered that there are two types of food allergies: *fixed* and *cyclical.* A fixed allergy is one that you acquire early in life or, for all practical purposes, are born with. So far, we are unable to offer any relief from fixed food allergies, except to caution the individual to stay away from the offending food. Fortunately, fixed allergies probably account for only 10 percent of a food-allergic person's total food reactions. The prognosis is better for cyclical allergies. These are food sensitivities that result from an individual's overexposing himself to a specific food. If you have difficulties with food, cyclical allergies will probably account for the other 90-percent of your food intolerances. Cyclical allergies were Jonathan's problem.

Management of cyclical allergies is based on the phenomenon that led you to acquire them in the first place. Since it is generally accepted that cyclical food allergies result from excessive exposure to a specific food or foods, the thought is that you can eliminate the allergy by abstaining from these reactive foods for a period of time. This allows your body the opportunity to recover from its attempt to cope with the allergy. It takes it off emergency status, so to speak, and makes it possible for it to return to its normal functions. After the appropriate abstinence period you can go back to eating your previously allergic foods, but only occasionally. Obviously it would be foolhardy to reinstate the food in the same amounts that caused the allergy in the first place.

For most people the food desensitization period takes a minimum of three months. Although some foods may be innately more irritating than others—pepper would seem to be naturally more irritating than a plain baked potato, for example—it appears to be more the frequency of exposure, rather than the kind of food or quantity ingested, that leads to the development of a food sensitivity. Thus, in the complex world of food allergies, food intolerance doesn't necessarily correlate with the quantity of food, but with how frequently the person eats it. Additionally, an individual with a low tolerance may experience a reaction from a tiny snack of the food to which he is sensitive, whereas someone else might tolerate a larger exposure before experiencing a reaction. The point is that food sensitivities vary among people, and it is your own reactions which you must observe, not those of someone else with a seemingly similar problem. Logically, the fundamental challenge in managing your food allergies is to determine what food you're allergic to. Identifying your troublesome foods and developing a diet to avoid them can take you a long way toward controlling your MS.

It is a characteristic of our modern society that food is pushed and shoved into various products and configurations. Corn can come on the cob, although probably increasingly less often these days. Corn is found in cereals, in ice cream and cakes (as corn syrup), as corn oil, as cornstarch thickeners, as margarine, as batter on fried foods, as part of the curing syrup in meats, in beer, in toothpaste, and in the glue on your stamps. The additives and food mixtures that have become a way of life, especially if you eat a lot of canned and frozen food, can make it extraordinarily complicated to identify and then avoid the foods that cause you to react.

We obviously recognize wheat when it appears on the table as a slice of bread or a piece of cake. However, it can also show up in such diverse items as gravy and soy sauce. Wheat flour is mixed with a variety of breads, even those supposedly made from corn or rye or oat flour. Eggs pose their own problems because they are present—but not necessarily evident—as an emollient in many foods, including ice cream. Some people react only to egg whites, others to yolks. Milk has its own set of problems, especially powdered milk, which appears routinely in a great variety of prepared foods.

All of this provides a challenge, not only in avoiding foods once you've identified those that bother you, but in trying to determine the culprits in the first place. The most efficient strategy, both for testing and for developing an alternative diet, is to use only whole, unprocessed foods. They're cheaper and better for you anyway. That way you don't have to spend a lot of frustrating time wondering whether it was the packaged green beans that bothered you, or the "butter sauce" they were served with, or the preservative or food dye the manufacturer added to keep them green and fresh.

As with most medical conditions, there are specialists to help you determine your food sensitivities. With the help of an understanding physician and a few simple rules, however, you can accomplish the task yourself. But this is not something you can do in your spare time. Nor should it be attempted as a diversion to lighten a boring afternoon. If you tend to operate that way, you might better check yourself into one of the clinical ecology clinics and have a specialist help.

In either case, there are a few essentials you will need—

patience, determination, and the ability to concentrate on detail and record it. Ah, you say, I thought there were easy ways to do it—like smearing my skin with tomatoes or apple sauce and watching the bumps rise. Unfortunately, both conventional allergists and food allergy specialists agree that skin tests for food allergies have proved to be inconsistent and unreliable. There are two laboratory tests, however, that have been used to help diagnose food allergies. These are the radioallergosorbent (RAST) test and the Cytotoxic Blood Test. In the former you will need to donate a sample of fresh blood, which the laboratory will scrutinize for evidence of antibodies to various foods. In the Cytotoxic Blood Test the blood sample is evaluated for white blood cell reaction to a variety of food extracts. Both tests have the advantage that they allow a variety of foods to be tested with only one blood sample. On the other hand, they have liabilities and, although popular, have proven not to be very helpful. Many reactions to foods appear in the absence of antibodies. Consequently, although accurate when the test is positive, this fact limits the number of foods that can be diagnosed with the RAST test and thus limits its usefulness. If you decide to submit to one of these tests, the best way to interpret the results is to accept those findings which indicate you are allergic to a food and go on to further testing of the foods the test says are safe.

These diagnostic tests aside, the test that is generally considered the most reliable for food allergies involves correlating food intake with the substantive appearance of symptoms, which—as we have seen—can range from diarrhea or constipation to dizziness and shortness of breath. Generally three systems have been applied to this effort. These are the escalation diet, the elimination diet, and the rotary diversified diet.

THE ESCALATION DIET

The Escalation Diet is based on evaluating only one food at a time, adding back foods only after you are sure of your reaction to them. You start by eating a single food for four to seven days and observe your reactions. After you have noted all your symptoms, you add another food, eating only your two foods for another four days, again noting any symptoms. This process is continued until you have tested all the foods you regularly eat. Orlanda Brown used a variation of this approach in detecting her allergies. There are, however, some difficulties with this system, which you should be aware of. For example, if you are an individual with a low food tolerance, repeated exposure to a food during the test period might cause you to become sensitized to a food that had previously caused you no difficulty. Also, there is obviously a certain monotony in eating the same food day after day for the two months or so that it would take to complete the test. This could result in the development of a craving for a food that hasn't yet been tested, thus compromising the trial.

THE ELIMINATION DIET

The elimination diet works somewhat in reverse. It is actually a two-step process. First you evaluate groups of foods, and then you go on to test individual foods from the groups that caused you to react. Although you may have not been aware of it, foods with similar characteristics are identified as belonging to certain food groups. Thus, when you test *legumes*, for example, your choice would include peanuts, soybeans, and something called tragacanth gum. Testing the apple group would allow you to select apples, pears, or quince. Even fish and meat are classified in groups. Decapods, for example, include crab, crayfish, lobster, prawns, and shrimp. Each group is tested for a two-week period, and the procedure is the same: you record any symptoms that appear as a result of eating that food group. Your goal is to identify classes of foods that might bother you and the others that you can classify as safe. After you've run through all the groups you have to go back and test the individual foods in each group that caused you trouble, thereby identifying the exact foods to avoid. One very practical advantage to this system is that it allows you some variety in what you eat during the test.

THE ROTARY DIVERSIFIED DIET

The rotary diversified diet is actually a modified elimination diet. It was developed to compensate for the mechanism that allows food allergies to go undetected in the first place—the phenomenon of masking. As we have seen, both fixed and cyclic allergic reactions may be hidden by overeating the offending food. Continued ingestion of a particular food keeps the allergy at a subclinical level so you don't realize your body is reacting. If you abstain from eating a food for at least four days, but not more than twelve, when you do eat that food again, symptoms are more apt to be readily apparent. You have unmasked your allergy. These symptoms will go away if you continue to abstain from the offending food a while longer; just how long is a function of your tolerance and level of addiction. Using the rotary diversified diet to unmask your food allergies is perhaps the most efficient and reliable system to determine the foods to which you're allergic.

However you choose to determine your allergies, it is important that you keep excellent records. You will have to note very carefully what you eat and the symptoms that may result. It is also helpful if you include such miscellaneous information as the time of day at which you take your meals, the size of your food portions, the time interval between ingestion of the food and the appearance of the symptoms, and any relative difference in symptoms as the days of the tests go on. One extremely important aspect of your record-keeping is that you record your information in a legible and organized fashion. You will be looking for patterns between the foods you eat and the symptoms you experience, so you will want to select a system for organizing your material so that it's readily retrievable.

Without doubt, the consummate record-keeper is Peter

Samuels. Peter started keeping detailed records when he began treatment at the university hospital. His journal consisted primarily of data on his MS symptoms and his reaction to the various types of treatment he received, although he also made it a point to make notes of his emotions and his psychological state of mind at the time. These experiences prepared him for keeping his food allergy journal.

Peter explains:

"You have to watch a lot of things that at first you wouldn't even think about. If you have eaten some kind of packaged or prepared food (which you'll soon learn is not worth it), you should include the brand name in your notes and perhaps a list of the ingredients as they appear on the package. A mistake that a lot of people make is that they list only the main foods at a meal. You have to describe everything—the butter on your toast, the pickle you had with your sandwich, the couple of potato chips you downed before dinner. You also have to list all the things you drink during the day, including water. It may seem time-consuming at first, but it's nothing compared to having to go back and try to reconstruct your meals because you've had an attack and are trying to trace its origins.

"I also found it helpful to jot down my activities for the day, so that I would know if I had inadvertently exposed myself to something else that might set me off. So far, I haven't found anything that bothers me but food. However, I like to give myself a chance in case someday I run into something I can't explain. Sometimes it may take a day or more for a food to produce its reaction, although most symptoms from food appear promptly. So it may take awhile for you to figure out which food caused the problem. Additionally, you may have to go back over a food more than once before deciding positively about it. Thus, the more detailed your records are, the easier it is to trace your problem."

Through his records, Peter determined that he routinely reacted to cane sugar. His MS got worse and he became short-tempered and irritable.

"Sometimes it takes three days for my emotions to settle down. I became irritable and intolerant of any unpredictable

behavior on the part of the children or my wife, even myself. You can use a known effect such as this to help you uncover something that you might have inadvertently eaten. If I get unreasonably angry with someone in the family or at work, for instance, I will start thinking back about what I've eaten for the last three or four days. Perhaps somehow I got into some sugar without even realizing it. If in my records I find something that I know has bothered me before, or if I notice that I've started eating a lot of a food I'd previously ignored, I'll immediately suspect it and cut it out, at least for a month. Then sometimes, just for the hell of it, I'll go back and try it again to see if I get a reaction. I do this especially if the suspected food is something I like.

"The aspect of the sugar business that's interesting is that when I was in college I was pretty good at sports. I was an especially mean son-of-a-gun on the football field. Looking back on it, I used to eat a lot of candy, actually anything that was loaded with sugar. It's kind of scary. I owe my football career to sugar."

So successful was Peter in using his food diary to identify his allergies that he didn't hesitate when a friend came to him complaining about a problem. Peter's friend was an executive in one of the town's major industries, who prided himself on his ability to concentrate and quickly assimilate complicated technical information. Gradually he began to notice that he was bothered by a ringing in his ears that became so intense that it distracted him from his reading. Not being one to tolerate such a problem needlessly, he made the rounds of the physicians in town, none of whom could determine the cause of the ringing. Still the problem persisted.

After watching this frustrating scenario unfold, Peter suggested to his friend that he might be reacting to something he ate. Peter instructed his friend to clean out his system by fasting for four days and then set him to work observing his symptoms. During the cleaning-out period the man's symptoms disappeared. Then, as he began adding back his regular foods one or two at a time, the ringing gradually returned.

During the testing he had identified gluten and wheat products and corn as his primary allergies. He discovered that his sensitivity to corn was so intense that the corn syrup in a teaspoon of ice cream would bother him for as long as four days. By avoiding the foods he couldn't tolerate, Peter's friend was able to resume his former pace.

THE PULSE TEST

Peter used the most reliable system for determining food allergies: the rotary diversified diet, combined with the pulse and niacin tests. The pulse test, originally described by food allergy pioneer Dr. Arthur Coca, is a simple method whereby you measure your pulse before a meal and at three intervals after you eat. It is routinely the case that a food to which you are allergic will cause your pulse to rise because it puts stress on your body.[1]

To use the pulse test, you first must establish a baseline for your pulse rate. You do this by taking your pulse before you get out of bed in the morning. A pre-rising pulse for the majority of people will usually be between 55 and 69 beats per minute. It is generally recommended that you take your pulse before you eat and three times after each meal, once at 30 minutes, once at 60, and then again at 90 minutes. You should also take your pulse just before you go to bed at night. Altogether, this would mean that you would be taking and recording your pulse a minimum of 14 times per day. If your pulse rises significantly after eating, you can assume that an allergic stress is being created by one or more of the food you've eaten.

You should equip yourself with a watch that has a second hand and sit quietly for five minutes before you start counting. The easiest place to find your pulse is at the artery in your wrist. To take your pulse, you simply count the beats for a *full* 60 seconds as measured by the second hand of your watch or clock. If you can't detect your pulse, you can use a stethoscope and listen to your heartbeat instead. Although there are a number of pulse meters on the market, they are inadequate for food testing because they estimate the pulse rate per minute on the basis of counting for only a few seconds. As we shall learn, variation of counts by only a few beats may be significant in determining your allergies, so a pulse rate estimate on a count for only 10 or fifteen seconds may result in significant error.

Assuming that you don't have an infection or haven't recently been exposed to any allergic food or other such substance, your *resting* pulse at any time during the day should generally not rise more than 16 beats per minute above your initial pre-rising rate. Additionally, your maximum resting pulse, whenever it may occur during the day, should not vary more than two beats per minute from one day to the next if you have remained free of your allergic foods. Thus, you should be alert to any changes from day to day, and anything above two beats could indicate an allergic reaction to something you've eaten. Coca, in fact, maintains that, on any given day, a pulse that exceeds six beats above your normal maximum pulse rate suggests an allergic reaction.[2] So, for example, if a person finds that his maximum pulse rate during the day is only six beats above his morning pre-rising level, but then discovers that his pulse jumped another six beats after eating a particular food, this twelve beat increase above his pre-rising pulse would most probably indicate allergy. Coca also has found that a maximum resting pulse rate for non-allergic people almost never exceeds 84 beats per minute.[3] If yours does at any time during the day, except after exercise, you should start looking for your allergic foods. This would, of course, not be the case for someone who is suffering from cardiovascular disease or an endocrine, infectious, toxic, or other type of traumatic condition at the time of testing. Recording your pulse rate readings on a graph is an excellent aid in helping you determine your average minimum and maximum resting pulse and noting any suspicious rises above your average maximum level.

There is an alternative procedure you might also want to employ in the interest of becoming extremely precise in detecting your allergic foods. Instead of matching your post-meal rate to your daily minimum, you match it to your pre-meal rate. If after you've eaten, your pulse exceeds six beats over your pre-meal rate, you should suspect an allergic reaction. In using this technique, however, you must be careful to take your pulse in the same sitting position each time. The best rule is to sit up straight in a chair any time you take your pulse. It is also helpful to have a table handy on which you can keep your watch or clock and your record-keeping material.

THE NIACIN TEST

The niacin test requires that you take 100 milligrams of niacin one hour before eating. If during that hour you experience a reaction, you probably have eaten something at a previous meal to which you're allergic. The usual reaction occurs at five to thirty minutes after a meal at which you've eaten something to which you're sensitive. This reaction typically consists of flushing or redness of the skin, usually about the head and neck, although it may appear over the entire body. It may also include prickling and itching of the skin, a common accompaniment of dilated superficial blood vessels. The reaction itself is benign, causes no serious problems, and will gradually subside. Generally, however, the stronger the allergic reaction to the food, the stronger the niacin reaction will be. Most individuals will find that they react to niacin only with the ingestion of certain foods. Conversely, avoidance of foods, such as happens during fasting, is associated with a disappearance of the flushing reaction, usually within the first two to three days, despite taking niacin. If you were to find yourself flushing with every meal, you are probably continually eating something you don't tolerate. It is extremely important to use a brand of niacin that doesn't contain a binder, coating, dye, or any extraneous material to which you might be allergic. Corn-starch, for example, is commonly added as a binder. Ask your pharmacist to obtain a niacin for you that is free of cornstarch and other potential allergens. A brand of corn-free niacin is available in the appropriate 100 milligram tablets from U. S. V. Pharmaceutical Corp. in Tarrytown, New York. Your pharmacist should be able to order it for you.

Before you implement the rotary diversified allergy detection system, it will help to review the six food allergy questions we discussed in the last chapter. The answers to these questions regarding your favorite, and not-so-favorite, foods will help you start thinking about your potential food problems. The next step is to use your answers to develop a list of your potentially troublesome foods. You then can proceed to use the pulse and niacin tests, either separately or together, while eating your regular meals. Use the tests for three days to determine reactions after each meal or snack. During the three-day pulse and niacin tests, you can eat your regular foods; you will be watching particularly for flushing reactions to niacin as well as a change in your pulse rate. It's a good idea to test the niacin you use to determine if the niacin or one of its components affects your pulse rate. To do this, simply check your pulse after taking niacin by itself in the same manner as you would after eating a particular food. It is at this step that you should start to keep records. Obviously you would be watching particularly for symptoms from the foods you identified in your answers to the six questions, but you should carefully observe any reactions to other foods. It's important to remember to include the foods from your potential allergy list in your menu for those three days.

The next step is more complicated. You make another list, this time of all the foods eaten at the meals after which you experienced a pulse or niacin reaction. You then proceed to test each food separately in a mini-meal test, in which you again use the pulse and niacin tests. To complete the mini-meal test you prepare a supply of the foods you think might be bothering you and then test them, one by one: a small glass of milk, one slice of bread, a tablespoonful of sugar dissolved in water. Before each mini-meal, take your pulse, and then afterward, once at 30, 60, and 90 minutes, as well as taking your niacin one hour before eating each food item. It will be easier to isolate the specific foods that bother you because you will be ingesting them alone instead of combined in a meal. Plan three hours to complete each individual food test, which means that you will be able to complete approximately four tests in any given day, so you should set aside three to four days for this procedure. (You may only be able to allow one-half hour between taking niacin and testing the food.)

Your final step is to implement the rotary diversified diet. This may be preceeded by an optional fast of four or five days to get all the toxins out of your system. Or as an alternative, you may use a supplement such as Vivonex (Norwich-Eaton), a hypoallergenic nutritional formula. It is strongly recommended that this be accomplished with the help and guidance of a physician. During the fast or the use of Vivonex, you may feel worse for a few days due to withdrawal symptoms. On the other hand, you may find that symptoms such as headache, stomach pains, or emotional distress may ease during this time. After your fast you add back the individual foods, one at a time, to which you had a pulse or niacin reaction during the mini-meal test. If you are allergic to any one of these, you may immediately experience a very distinct reaction because the fasting period will cause you to lose a state of relative tolerance that you have developed to these allergic foods. These will be the withdrawal symptoms we talked about in our discussion of food allergies. During this time you should also be using the pulse and niacin tests to verify your symptoms. Throughout your testing procedures, you will need to use both the pulse and niacin tests, because the consistency of their reactions varies among food and among people.

Orlanda explains how she detected her food allergies. Her system was somewhat hit-or-miss, but because she was so diligent, she was able to identify the foods that bothered her. She started with observing her symptoms, which she then confirmed with the pulse and niacin tests.

"I started right in with a kind of modified escalation diet. I didn't do the three-day full-meal pulse and niacin tests or the mini-meal test. I would set up a week of possible menus. First I would have something like chicken and oranges for breakfast and see if I got a reaction. If I did, then I knew I'd have to test both foods individually. I suspected oranges because I had determined that I'm allergic to grapefruit and the two are in the same family. So my next step would be to try chicken at lunch, in combination with something I knew was safe— like rice. If I didn't react, then I knew my morning reaction was to the oranges. If I wanted to confirm my suspicions about oranges, I'd have them at dinner with the rice and chicken. If I reacted, then I knew positively that I couldn't eat oranges.

"You have to have a place to start, of course, and we started with the foods that I had eaten when I was sick—grapefruit and whole-wheat crackers—which I depended on when I thought I couldn't eat anything else. At first it was a real pain to go through all this; I mean baked potatoes for breakfast? But then I'd think back to when I was at school and feeling terrible. I remember there were times, at night especially, when I would have trouble getting my bearings relative to other things. I'd knock something off the dresser and wouldn't realize it until I got up in the morning and found it on the floor.

"It's true that it takes time and patience to determine which foods bother you, but I had been sick for so long without any hope of finding out what was the matter. So when I found out about food allergies I felt like I had no alternative but to go for it. I had gone to every kind of doctor there was, even an ear, nose, and throat specialist. Everyone kept telling me to calm down. I felt like one of those kids who is always jumping around. I would have calmed down if I could. Nobody knew how to help me do it. They just wanted me to stop being sick and 'act normal.'"

In using the pulse test to help determine your allergies, you should remember a number of guidelines. First of all, be practical. Don't take your pulse immediately after exercise, even if it's just walking, because you won't get an accurate reading. You should also not attempt the pulse test if you are ill with a cold or the flu or some other infection. Most normal people in good health, except for any possible food allergies, should have a pre-rising pulse of between 55 and 69 beats per minute or less. If, under normal circumstances, your pulse were to rise at least 16 beats above your pre-rising leval—or six beats above your average daily maximum rate—then it's likely you are allergic to something you've just eaten. When you use the pulse test, you are looking for variations in the rate over the entire day, rather than trying to match your rate to an absolute scale.

Additional factors can cause your pulse to rise, specifically airborne allergens such as dust, cosmetics such as hair spray, and health aids such as vitamins and toothpaste. If you have searched out and eliminated all your food allergens, but are still experiencing a rise in your pulse, then you will have to test yourself with other substances to which you are commonly exposed. Additionally, if you assemble your new allergen-free diet and still react, remember that sometimes a strong food allergen will hide one that is less potent, so that your reaction to the latter will appear until the former is eliminated from your diet. You might also consider that you may not have eaten all of your allergenic foods during the test period. A cyclical allergy to a food you have avoided eating for a while also may not cause a reaction because abstinence has reduced your sensitivity. If you substitute it for another food to which you know you're allergic, your previous sensitivity will return. As you gradually eliminate your allergic foods, you may notice a general decrease in your minimum and maximum pulse rates, which will mean that you'll have to adjust the pulse at which you recognize an allergic food. Generally, your pulse will be lower because you are eliminating the stress on your body that caused it to rise. If you keep careful records on your graph, you will immediately notice these differences and can adjust your testing accordingly.

Cindy Morse, for example, had developed a new diet and

was doing an excellent job of adhering to her new program, when suddenly she had an acute exacerbation of MS. She reviewed the foods she had eaten in the prior three days and satisfied herself that she hadn't purposefully or inadvertently eaten one of her troublesome ones. She and her husband then checked over their activities for the same time period. It didn't take long to pinpoint the potential problem—they had spent the afternoon the day before spreading fertilizer on their back lawn. Cindy believes it was the fertilizer that caused her attack. For two weeks after that she continued to be bothered by the MS, as the fertilizer soaked slowly into the grass.

SUMMARY

To recap, there are a few rather simple steps to follow in determining whether or not you're suffering from food allergies and what foods might be bothering you.

The first thing is to discuss this problem with your doctor, a doctor who can help in this process. He should be aware of your medical history and interested in what you're doing. Additionally, some individuals have been known to have dramatic reactions when they add back the foods they are allergic to after a period of abstinence. Although such reactions are usually not any more serious than a mild headache or an upset stomach, if this concerns you, be sure you enter the process in conjunction with your physician.

The Six Questions

As you meet with your doctor you should develop answers to the six questions about your food habits and preferences. From the answers to those questions you can then develop a list of foods that you should make sure to test. These will be the foods you eat most frequently, those to which you're fairly sure you're not allergic, and those you consider would be the hardest to give up. This is **List A,** your list of preliminary suspects.

The Pulse and Niacin Tests

You can now proceed to the pulse and niacin tests to check your regular diet. Eat as you usually do, but make sure that your meals contain all the foods on List A. It will help if you eliminate in-between-meal snacks because they will complicate the pulse-taking procedure. If you regularly eat a snack of some kind in the morning or afternoon or before you go to bed, include it in the test but eat it at the preceding meal. Take your pulse before you get out of bed each day, before each meal, and then 30, 60, and 90 minutes afterward. Take the niacin an hour before you eat and watch for the flushing reaction five minutes to an hour after the meal. List all foods you eat at each meal and note any special or unusual activities. Do this for three days. If you have any systemic symptoms such as fatigue, looseness of stool, dizziness, headache, constipation, etc., be very sure to note these in detail.

After the three days, take a look at your records, noticing where your pulse jumped and any meals after which you experience flushing. If you observe a reaction, take a look at the foods you ate at that meal or as snacks. List all the contents of these meals. This is **List B.** Remember all condiments and sauces.

The Mini-Meal Test

Now you can go on to the mini-meal test in which you will individually evaluate your suspected foods using the pulse and niacin tests and observing any other symptoms that might appear. Again you will be recording the food eaten and the pulse and niacin reactions. It is also helpful if you enter the quantity you ate of each food tested. You should repeat this until you run through all the foods on List B.

At the completion of the mini-meal test, list all those foods for which you confirmed a pulse or niacin response or to which you experienced some other reaction. This is **List C.** You're getting close.

The Rotary Diversified Diet

The purpose of the rotary diversified diet is to confirm the previous results of your mini-meal test and to test any other foods you might have missed because you didn't eat them during that test. Prior to starting the rotary diversified diet, you may want to fast for four or five days as described. For the remainder of this part of the test you will be sustaining yourself mainly on those foods you know are safe. You should pick a number of foods—broiled chicken or fish, for example; rice, a few vegetables—and resign yourself to eating them for a few weeks as you rotate in and out the foods you think are bothering you. There is also the alternative of sustaining yourself during this period on Vivonex as you would during the fast, but basically it is more practical if you simply eat the foods to which you haven't reacted. Start with the food at the top of List C and reintroduce it to your diet for one day, along with the other foods that should be nonreactive. Take your pulse in the usual manner before and after each meal. Be sure to also use niacin, and note any symptoms until you've tested all the foods on the list. If any one food caused significant symptoms, you should wait until the symptoms clear before you test another food. Otherwise you risk confusing the reactions. Depending on how many foods you're testing, plan on eating this way for three to four weeks.

Make a fourth list, **List D,** which will contain all the foods you've identified that caused a reaction during your tests. These are your major food allergies. You may find other foods or additives that cause you trouble, but for the moment, you know you should avoid the foods on List D. If, after being on your new diet for a while, you observe symptoms or have reason to suspect other foods, you should start the procedure again, continuing with the three-day pulse and niacin tests, the mini-meal test, and proceeding through the rotary diversified diet.

Initially, these testing procedures may seem a bit cumbersome, but keep in mind the importance of your results. As Peter Samuels says, *"There is absolutely nothing more dramatic than using these tests, especially monitoring your symptoms as you reinstate an allergenic food into your diet. You eat the food and you get a reaction. You don't eat it, you're symptom-free. What could be more simple than that?"*

8

DEVISING
YOUR DIET

Have you ever noticed that when someone finds himself stuck in a difficult situation those around him, in an effort to help, frequently fall back on the old saw of "keeping a stiff upper lip"? The thought seems to be that, if you can prevent yourself from falling into despair at your circumstances, you might be able to beat them. Perhaps this bit of folk wisdom is based on our national belief that, if you just try hard enough, you're bound to succeed, even against insurmountable odds.

Although there are an ample number of inspiring testimonials that this attitude does indeed produce results—just look at the origins of some of our presidents—the costs are often high. Conversely, if this course doesn't deliver, the result can be disillusionment, which may be more lethal than the actual failure. On the other hand, you should, of course, prioritize your challenges, and it must be admitted that changing your diet will not be the easiest thing in the world to accomplish. You are tampering here with one of your basic drives—the need for food—more powerful, the experts tell us, and more urgent than sex. Plus, change of any kind is difficult. We generally develop habits because, as the psychologists say, they provide some sort of "payoff." Practically speaking, that means that people don't often engage in behavior that doesn't "get them something." Rewards vary, of course, in kind and value, from public acknowledgment of one's capabilities to the negative attention sought by a naughty child.

In modifying your eating habits, you are struggling with the development of new behavior patterns—as well as learning new strategies for implementing them. You are also dealing with one of the most pleasurable of our civilized activities, the time spent at the table, with food, drink, and, hopefully, good company.

In your plan for change, your goal should be to develop a system for controlling your food allergies so you can, in turn, diminish the effects of multiple sclerosis.

Fundamentally, you must remember that, if you have a food allergy, you must not only change what you eat, but also alter your approach to food. Food will never again be a completely wanton source of pleasure. Not that for most people it ever has been, at least since we passed from the days of Henry VIII into the age of diabetes, atherosclerosis, and hypertension. You will probably never again be able to eat exactly what you want when you want, and the devil be damned. Because the devil won't be damned, you'll be uncomfortable and probably sick. The "up" side of all of this is that your food preferences are mostly learned. You are not born with a taste for corn on the cob with lots of butter and salt and pepper, or snails with garlic, or even a plain potato. Somewhere along the line you learned what you like.

Throughout our lifetimes, we are all exposed to different kinds of foods. Some we find agreeable, others (like creamed chipped beef on toast) probably not as much so. We all have tasted, and probably will continue to taste, food in different types of circumstances and under varying conditions, factors that will influence our perception of whether we enjoy it or not. There are probably thousands of sailors and former sailors in this country who dislike creamed chipped beef for just that reason—they had too much of it in the wrong place at the wrong time.

So, if you have to eliminate a food from your diet, or perhaps eat it infrequently, you can replace it. What you substitute may be something you'll eventually come to enjoy a great deal. There's a vast world of raw foodstuffs out there, along with thousands of recipes for combining them, and most of us will never get a chance to scratch the surface. Although it may seem impossible that anything could replace your favorite coconut cake or your sister's lemon meringue pie, such miracles have been known to happen. Especially if you remember the payoff—you'll be healthier.

Going cold turkey on a favorite food, with all the feeling-sorry-for-yourself that can go along with it, is not the only strategy for coping with food allergies. In fact, it is undoubtedly not the optimal one. If you get into substituting something "safe" for something to which you're allergic, and if you eat the new food in the same way as you did the old—*compulsively*—you'll run the risk of developing new allergies. The most effective solution is to adopt new eating habits. In place of the conventional battle of willpower against taste buds (in which willpower often loses), let's examine some possibilities for developing new ways of eating.

Actually, if we were to take a close look at our national eating habits, we would have to admit that we've become a nation of food abusers. Not that we're alone in this; the hectic pace of life in the industrialized world has turned a unique opportunity into a sorry liability. Probably at no other time in history—except perhaps during the Roman Empire, when the quest for unusual foods became a national mania and a rich man's hobby—have so many different foods been so available to so many people. Modern methods of agriculture and transportation have made it possible for people in the northern United States to eat oranges from Florida in the winter, tomatoes from California year-round, and fresh pineapple from Hawaii, while people in California feast on fresh Maine lobster and Maryland soft-shell crab. We're far removed from the days when it was necessary to keep a cow out back in order to enjoy beef or a chicken coop for a fryer and fresh eggs. Additionally, a new class of experts—the chef/gourmets—have attempted to expand our horizons about what is edible. Still, we persist in our habits of eating the same old things.

Our abuse of food, in fact, has become so serious that we might be said to have come to disregard it entirely. "Oh," you react, "that's impossible in this nation of fast-food chains and huge supermarkets. Food is everywhere. We are obsessed with food." Actually we are probably more obsessed with eating than with food. It has become a kind of mindless national pastime. What do the fast-food chains offer that could possibly be categorized as reasonably interesting or healthy? Beef on a bun and potatoes or chicken encased in batter and grease—not much variety or subtlety there. Perhaps it is not happenstance that our most common food allergies are those to red meat, milk, wheat, potatoes, corn, and eggs. All are abundantly available on almost every street corner, and some have been elevated as symbols of status— the sirloin steak, for example. If a man can serve his family steak, or order one whenever he likes at a restaurant, he may, by some standards, be said to have "made it." Whoever heard of impressing your friends with some delicately poached sole—despite the fact that in many American cities, a piece of fish now costs more than a slice of beef? Our most commonly eaten foodstuffs come at us constantly in snack food form—french fried potatoes, ice cream cones, hamburgers; eggs for breakfast or anytime—scrambled, fried, over easy, or hard-boiled. How would a coffee shop survive without them? If a fast-food chain takes a chance and serves fish, then it's coated with a batter that makes it taste like a cross between a hamburger and a french fry, which could be the intent.

All of this is meant to provide you with some perspective on food. People tend to feel bad when they have to give up something, especially if it's pleasurable. But what we've done with food, if you really think about it, is to make it boring. Expanding your food horizons as you attempt to control your allergies can actually become an exciting experience if you give it a chance. There are lots of good things to eat out there that we don't even think about, but we tend to suspect many of them. Confronted with the option of trying something new, people have been known to respond with questions like "Millet? What is millet? Where do you get it? Aren't health food stores for freaks? What is barley? I think my mother used it in soup. I never heard of kale, but it sounds like something slimy."

As you adjust your diet, try to keep this thought in mind: you were not necessarily born with the birthright of steak and potatoes for dinner or eggs and bacon for breakfast, nor did your body intend for you to gorge yourself on ice cream three times a day. All pervasive food company giants and their advertising aside, you have your own good health to think of. Start small and gradually expand your horizons. Try not to be compulsive; give your taste buds a chance to adjust and your emotions time to mourn the loss of your favorite foods. They'll be gone for good, with all your "tears" shed.

To aid people with food allergies, the rotary diversified diet has been developed. We spoke about it in the last chapter and showed you how you can use it to help diagnose your food allergies. We like to think of it as an expanded diet because it calls for you to eat a wide variety of foods, but none frequently enough to expose yourself to developing additional cyclical allergies. Your first job is to familiarize yourself with the food families we discussed in the last chapter. Although at first it will take a little paper rattling to get everything straight, it doesn't take long before utilizing this system becomes second nature. You can be as organized or as casual as you want, as long as you feel comfortable in absorbing and using the information. Take your time and do the following methodically.

Rule 1: Maintain four days between specific foods, two days between families.

The food groups are essential to the rotary diversified diet, and two rules are essential in establishing your menus. First you have to allow two days between eating foods from the same group; second, you cannot eat the same food any more often than once every four days. This means that if on day one of your new routine you ate an apple, you could not eat a pear until day three, because pears are in the same family.

Equally as important, you couldn't eat another apple until day five. A complete description of the food groups is available in Chapter 10.

If it happens to be berry season, and you've loaded up on the rose family, you could eat one of them every other day—strawberries on day one, bananas on day two (bananas are a different family), raspberries on day three, (the rose family again), oranges on day four, strawberries on day five, and a banana again on day six. Just don't repeat strawberries until the fifth day or have a banana again until day six.

You can mix foods from different families on the same day. Suppose you want to have a tangerine for breakfast and strawberries for dinner on the same day. That would be OK, as long as on the next day you don't have anything from either the rose or citrus family. The day after that, however, you could have an orange for breakfast and boysenberries for dinner. You want to be careful not to use up too many options in one day or, worse, in one dish, like a fruit cocktail. It's much easier in practice than it sounds here.

There are more than nine fruit families, so you wouldn't have trouble rotating them. But you do have to know which fruit falls into which family. Vegetables are spread over more than a dozen different families; herbs are found in about four families, spices in as many as six. All of which provides you the opportunity for variety that you wouldn't have known about if you had opted for willpower and the stiff-upper-lip method. There are thirteen fish families and an additional sixteen types of fish that have no families, so that with certain kinds of fish you wouldn't have to worry about maintaining the day in between. For example, you could eat swordfish one day, whitefish the next, and a piece of ocean perch the next. If you wanted to eat tuna and mackerel, however, you'd have to skip a day in between because they're in the same family; likewise lobster and shrimp.

Animal protein tends to fall into the same pattern, single families. There are five separate bird families, for example: (1) chicken, pheasant, and quail; (2) duck and goose; (3) grouse; (4) guinea hen; and (5) turkey. On the red meat side, the bovines are considered one family—beef, buffalo, lamb, and goat. Don't laugh; both buffalo and goat are very tasty, and if you can get them, it would be possible to rotate them with the more conventional beef and lamb. Other mammals such as pork arc thcir own families.

In implementing your rotary diversified diet, you will need to pay particular attention to sauces, seasonings, and the cooking process. If you have a sensitivity to corn, for example, you'd have to watch for the day you eat corn on the cob to make sure you don't use corn oil on your salad the next day or a margarine made from corn oil. If wheat is your downfall, then macaroni one day would obviously rule out a sandwich the next, unless you knew you had a bread made with 100-percent nonwheat flour. Bread, of course, is never a good selection because it is a mixture of multiple ingredients and thus increases your chance of reacting. More importantly, you'd also have to watch out for gravies, sauces, or soups thickened with wheat flour. If you were eating at home, you might substitute potato starch or rice flour and then not have to worry about the macaroni you ate the day before.

Cereals are the most difficult family to work with because they're all-inclusive. Barley, corn, millet, oats, wheat, rice, rye, and wild rice are all in the cereal family, along with a few you probably don't have to worry about—bamboo, sorghum, sugarcane, and triticale. As a cereal substitute, you really have only buckwheat. If your problem is the gluten in the grain, rather than the whole grain itself, you could rotate the gluten-containing cereals with the two that are gluten-free—rice and millet. Thus, on a gluten-sensitivity diet, you could have oatmeal for breakfast one day and brown rice the next, then rye crackers the next, muffins made with millet flour the next, a noncereal dish such as eggs on the next, and finally, oatmeal on the next, which would be the fifth day. If you were allergic to wheat, your rotation would go something like this: oatmeal on day one, buckwheat cereal on day two, whole grain cereal (read the label to verify ingredients) on day three, a noncereal-type dish on day four, and then back to your oatmeal on day five.

Dairy products are essentially their own family and require special attention. If you eat a carton of plain yogurt on day one, that's it for dairy products for the next four days. This would include butter, cream, whipped cream, ice cream, cottage cheese, and any other kind of hard or soft cheese. Ice cream and flavored yogurts are mixtures of several ingredients and ideally should be avoided. In cases such as this, where one day wipes out the next four, on your allotted day you might be tempted to load up on as much of the product as you can. Indeed, some specialists say that you may combine foods from within one family in a day—milk on your buckwheat in the morning, cottage cheese for lunch, and a glass of milk at dinner. Their opinion is based on the fact that it is the frequency with which a food is eaten, not the amount, that effects the allergic reaction. Others would caution that individuals with a tendency toward allergy should be practical and monitor the amount of any given food they eat, preferably eating any food in relatively small quantities. They indicate that the individual who observes symptoms after eating a food should definitely cut down and perhaps even avoid that food for awhile. In the case of dairy products, if you really have trouble weaning yourself from the habit of, say, cereal and milk for breakfast, try one of the milk substitutes, goat's milk or soy milk. Either one will probably destroy your yearning altogether and let you get down to being more creative about your first meal of the day.

In addition to developing a rotating menu you will have to consider your food preparation. The general rule is: the simpler the better. Meat is better broiled, baked, or steamed without sauces and coatings; use spices instead. You should avoid a lot of frying because it takes oil, which will both complicate your menu and—if you use it too often—expose you to the risk of developing an additional allergy. If you are allergic to corn, shrimp fried in corn oil one night, or with cornmeal breading, would knock out your corn oil salad dressing tomorrow, or your popcorn, or corn on the cob, or cornbread, anything thickened with cornstarch, and ice cream sweetened with corn sugar. There are a number of different oils on the market that you could rotate for both variety and taste. Besides soybean oil, there are also olive oil, walnut oil, peanut oil, safflower oil, and sunflower seed oil, some of which are generally available in supermarkets, others in specialty food stores.

Rule 2: Eat *simply;* buy fresh, unprocessed food as much as possible. Cook it simply without a lot of additional sauces.

Your vegetables are better eaten raw or steamed or boiled; they'll taste better and be better for you both nutritionally and allergywise. Potatoes and other types of vegetables such as squash can be baked, as long as they don't end up coated with gobs of butter and sour cream. Fruits are best eaten fresh or poached. The obvious caution here is to stay away from prepared foods, especially canned goods, boxed mixtures, and the frozen items with special sauces and toppings, which can contain food substances you're allergic to, as well as food additives and synthetic flavors and colors. Once you become familiar with your supermarket's produce section you'll discover that fresh vegetables need no additional sauces, flavor additives, or dyes to make them appealing. One carton of frozen "Chinese-style vegetables in special sauce" can eliminate three or four food families in one dish: first the vegetables (green peppers, broccoli, garlic, onions, and peas); then the peanut oil in which they were stir-fried; the soy sauce; and perhaps flour or cornstarch used to thicken the sauce. Add to this any flavor enhancers such as MSG and a preservative to give it a longer shelf life, and you've got quite a number of substances to work around. It would be better if you picked one fresh vegetable, took it home, steamed it and added a little lemon, margarine, or garlic salt.

Rule 3: Be diligent about checking ingredients; don't guess.

Preparing your food from scratch at home may seem time-consuming at first, but think of it as time better spent than loitering around supermarkets reading labels. Not that you shouldn't do that. If you have to buy prepared foods, checking labels is essential; but your goal should be to go home with the fresh goods and leave the boxes and cans of overprocessed stuff to people who aren't conscientious about their health. "The simpler, the better" also applies to the variety of food you consume in any given day. A mixed salad for lunch could leave you vegetableless for days, whereas sliced tomatoes for dinner one evening would leave cucumbers for the next and broccoli for a side dish.

In planning your rotary diet, try to develop a second sense. It will pay off in the long run. Janet Myerson discovered this immediately.

"I turned out to be allergic to dairy products. Milk seemed easy enough to avoid, but look at the rest of the list: buttermilk, cream, sour cream, ice cream, yogurt, and everything with nonfat dry milk, which is a lot, from those diet concoctions to hot chocolate. It also means no baked products, no sauces or gravies made with milk, no creamed soups, and no cheese, except goat cheese, which I finally tried, and it turned out to be quite good. Also, no pudding, custard, or omelets unless I know what went into them. I'm especially careful when I'm out to dinner. I have a friend who discovered she's allergic to eggs. She has to watch out for things I never have thought about—baked goods, pancakes, some kinds of pasta, and some salad dressings. When we go out together, we usually take our own dressing because I'm also allergic to corn, and sometimes they make their dressings with corn oil."

Wheat-sleuthing is one of the toughest. Orlanda Brown eliminated her wheat crackers and grapefruit immediately. She then had to learn how to avoid her mother's coffee cakes—*"I take long walks. At first I would sneak up to it and grab a few walnuts off the top, but that was a little too close for comfort. When the craving for something gets particularly bad, I just go out and walk for half an hour. I never ate much bread—except for rolls—so that wasn't too much of a problem. My mom wanted me to try rye bread, but most kinds have wheat flour in them. I mean, the things you learn. Sometimes fried food has corn coating, sometimes wheat, so I just stay away from the fried stuff. It's better for my complexion anyway. Oh, yeah, whiskey pie, that was another real temptation, but I got over it. Some days I feel sorry for myself. But who needs a piece of whiskey pie every day?"*

Rule 4: Don't cheat; a little slip on your rotation can throw off the entire plan.

Corn probably runs second to wheat in terms of difficulty in ferreting out its presence in foods, because cornstarch is used as a thickener in so many foods, from catsup to pudding, in all kinds of creamed dishes, even in toothpaste and cough syrup. One food allergist lists 150 generally available products containing corn. Corn is in dextrose, for example, which is a common ingredient in a variety of prepared foods. If you're affected by cane sugar, you also have to be extremely diligent. Sugar is everywhere, often listed on the ingredient information as sucrose, which is white sugar. Because sugar is used in so many foods, even vegetables if they're frozen or canned, you must become a real sleuth when you stumble into the frozen or canned food sections. Even something as seemingly uncomplicated as fruit juice might throw off your system. If, for example, you picked up a brand that was sweetened with cane sugar and followed it the next day with another juice or a prepared product that also contains sugar, you would be breaking your rotation. It may seem easy enough to give into the temptation of sneaking just a little bit, using the rationale that a small amount can't hurt. Remember, however, that with food allergies, the little bit on a regular basis can be worse than the occasional big binge. Frequent exposure, no matter how minuscule the portion, can do you in.

Rule 5: Do not implement the rotary diversified diet until you've cleared your allergic foods—don't skimp on the three-month desensitization period.

Rule 6: Plan carefully and keep records. It will save you time in the long run.

Having assembled your knowledge about food groups and compared it with your knowledge of the foods that bother you, your next task is to avoid those foods for the three to four months it will take to desensitize yourself. The period of time it takes for your body to recover from the effects of attempting to metabolize irritating food will vary with the individual. This is called the *refractory stage;* it's a healing process that generally begins about three weeks after you've stopped eating the allergy-producing foods. This doesn't mean you should try to reintroduce an irritating food at three weeks. The healing process has just begun. If, after the three months, you attempt to reintroduce a food and experience a reaction, you must go off the food again for another three months. You may find that you can eat the formerly troublesome food but not as often as every four days, as the rotary diversified diet specifies. This is something you must experiment with yourself. If you get a reaction from a frequent exposure, then simply try the food once every five days or perhaps once a week. Whatever you do, don't try to kid yourself or laugh off symptoms. You'll only end up recreating your former allergic reaction—and then have to start all over again.

SUMMARY

Briefly, let's review the rotary diversified diet, remembering that while it is an excellent system for living with cyclical food allergies, it will not solve the problem of a fixed allergy. For that, you have no alternative but to avoid the offending substance. Since 90-percent of our allergies are cyclic, however, you will be able to live well on the rotary diet and still control your allergies.

The Desensitization Period

You must avoid your primary allergens for three months. During that time you will have time to do your long-suffering bit, complaining about never being able to have a dish of ice cream or a piece of pie. All this will come to an end, however, if you're diligent and patient. To help you in this process you might want to try substituting foodstuffs. This can also aid you in diversifying your rotary diet once you desensitize yourself. Orlanda Brown, for example, tired of her baked potatoes and rice for breakfast, learned how to make rice flour muffins. Her biggest challenge was finding the flour, which her mother finally discovered in a health food store.

There are milk substitutes, although they get mixed reviews as to taste. If you want to try goat's milk, be sure to avoid the canned variety and buy fresh. Instead of soybean milk, which necessarily tastes like soybeans and may contain additives, you might try an old medieval specialty—nut milk made from cashews or almonds. You boil the nuts in water and then run the mixture through a food processor or blender and refrigerate. You can also grind nuts and mix with dried fruit and use the mixture as a cereal substitute for breakfast. It takes a while to chew through a bowl of chopped nuts, however, so you'll have to allow an extra ten minutes for breakfast. Janet Myerson's mother-in-law prowled the specialty food stores for wheat-free flour, soybean milk, millet, and buckwheat. She also found a number of catalogues that helped her locate some of the more difficult items Janet used.

Use the desensitization period to plan for your rotary diet. Organize your food families by categories of foods—all the fruit families together, all the vegetable families, herbs, spices, meat, and fish. This will help you when you get to menu planning. You'll be able to look at your lists and make choices easily. Since you're going to rotate your menu, you don't have to include special notations about foods you know you're allergic to. Your business now is simply to create a wonderful food regimen for yourself.

The Rotary Diversified Diet

Go through all the food groups and identify those foods you've never tasted, along with those you know but aren't sure where to buy them. Your objective during this time is to try new foods and select sources of supply for those that might be difficult to find. Not all the foods you've missed thus far in your life will require a trip down some exotic back alley. A lot of them are in your supermarket; you probably have never noticed them. If you are a regular customer, chances are your manager will stock something you need if he doesn't presently carry it. If you have difficulty locating a specific food or food substitute, consult the specialized food resource sections included in the allergy cookbooks listed in the appendix. You might want to make a list of difficult-to-obtain foods and their sources. Such a list might also include an inventory of your supply of these kinds of foods so that you don't end up frazzled from running out of something that's essential.

As you try new foods, add comments to your list, so you know why you liked or didn't like something. You may want to try it again later, or you may notice that the new food goes particularly well with something you already like. If you have any trouble with your record-keeping—difficulty with reading or writing—or if your memory isn't as sharp as you'd like it to be, ask someone to help you. This could be a sympathetic person who is interested in your project. Orlanda asked her mother to help her, and both ended up enjoying their new foods and cooking methods. Or you might choose someone who's having difficulty adjusting to your disease. Suzanne might have used this system to educate her husband about her condition and perhaps increase his understanding.

You should also identify the auxiliary equipment or materials you'll need for your diet—cooking oils, for example, margarines and additional spices. Perhaps you might buy yourself some new cooking utensils. Some nonstick pans will be useful, so you don't have to use oil when you're baking or frying. If you need it, get yourself a magnifying glass to read labels and start collecting allergy cookbooks. Your library will have some, and there is a handy list in the back of this book. Make up your own list of substitutions so you're ready, and have them at hand for planned use and your occasional emergencies.

The Menu

Now you are ready to lay out your first week of meals. It might be easier if you set up a page of your notebook as a calendar for a week and mark off the days into six sections: one for each of your main meals and one for each of three snacks if you eat them. But don't kid yourself about this; you will have to keep track of what you eat in between meals or you run the risk of thwarting the whole plan. This means all beverages as well. To start with, follow your usual meal preferences. If you like juice and cereal and milk and a beverage for breakfast, plan your first breakfast that way, listing the kind of juice you're going to have, the cereal, and the milk. If you squeeze your own juice or can buy the fresh-squeezed kind as Janet does, then you don't have to worry about added sugar. If you'd rather have an egg and toast, plan it that way, making sure you note the kind of bread you're using for your toast (and its ingredients) and how the egg is going to be cooked. Proceed in a similar fashion for the rest of your day. When you finish with day one, do the same with day two. You might even want to write down on paper what you would usually have that day, then look at your food family list, do a little creative thinking, and make your substitutions.

If you follow your usual food patterns for the first week and rotate your choices, your new menu won't seem as strange to you. As you become more experienced, you might want to try some new patterns for breakfast. If you run out of cereals, for example, try rice for breakfast—brown rice with milk and cinnamon is especially good. Or try something unusual like fish.

If you don't do the cooking in the family, consult the person who does. Explain your menu and see if it can be integrated with the family meals. You might also want to help your cook prepare some special meals and freeze them so you can have them on hand. It is also wise to take the time to sit down with your family and explain to them what you're doing. Be firm about your need for their support. Almost everyone likes to eat, and you have a right to be able to eat things that taste good and minimize the threat of illness.

Test yourself to determine how much planning you're comfortable with. Do you want to plan for two weeks and then just start the menu again? Or would you rather plan for a whole month? These things are up to you—just as long as the planning gets done. Be sure to leave room on your menu to indicate any adverse reactions. If you do experience symptoms as a result of a meal, review the foods you ate, identify the culprit, and test it four days later at a single meal. If you continue to experience symptoms, abstain from the food for another three months before putting it back in rotation.

Throughout this process, it's important for you to remember that it will take you a little more time to buy and cook your food. You will have to think more about what you eat, especially in the beginning. But you'll be reinforced for the time you spend on this worthwhile project. You'll have the fun of discovering new and interesting foods and cooking techniques. You'll also feel better. Most of all, it certainly beats the alternative of having MS and spending your time doing nothing about it.

9

STAYING ON
YOUR DIET

We Americans have appropriated one of Britain's most famous exports. We buy books about him and flock to see him on the screen. Not only is he honest and upright, successful at what he does, cosmopolitan, urbane and handsome, and fit; he is also consistent. A man like this would certainly be concerned about his food. So we understand when James Bond has "the usual" and orders his breakfast: bacon, two eggs, toast, marmalade, and coffee. Every day the same thing. Consistency aside, one hopes Mr. Bond doesn't have a predisposition to allergy.

Although consistency may be a virtue in some areas, we have already seen that in the matters that concern us here it can be a crucial, detrimental factor. Regardless of your perception of your own regularity or spontaneity regarding food, you need to spend some time evaluating your eating patterns. Your observations will be a primary element in your plan to implement a new dietary system successfully. The self-knowledge you gain through this process protects you against backsliding as well as the anxiety and frustration that can thwart your efforts to control your allergies and alleviate the symptoms of MS.

In the preceding chapters we have talked at length about the necessity of keeping records. At first it might seem that we are wasting valuable time with paper and pencil rather than getting down to business. But as Hamlet said, "Though this be madness, yet there is method in 't."

Psychologists and psychological therapists routinely use record-keeping as a crucial element in programs designed for people desiring to implement a lifestyle change. Although the system in its entirety is too complicated to present in detail here, a number of the required strategies are useful. In fact, some elements of these programs have been implemented intuitively by MS patients who have established successful plans for living with their food allergies.

In psychological language this approach is referred to as *self-management*. It means that the individual himself, as opposed to the psychologist or therapist, is responsible for developing and implementing his own program. This system depends heavily on the individual's commitment to provide information about himself and his current behavior so that he can plan what he would like to change and how he will go about doing it. The record-keeping that is essential to self-management techniques also provides constant feedback about his progress by requiring the person to carefully monitor his efforts to implement his new behavior.[1]

Modern psychology is divided into two primary schools of thought. One views an individual's behavior as being a function of his recollected past experiences and seeks an understanding of how that may affect his current actions. The goal is to alleviate unresolved conflicts from his past so he may achieve a healthy adjustment to his present circumstances. This is referred to as the *psychoanalytical approach* and depends heavily on an ongoing relationship between the therapist and patient.

The second school of modern psychological thought is *behaviorism*, which considers observed behavior to be the starting point for therapy. In a sense it seeks to shortcut the "why" of behavior to examine its suitability to the circumstances in which the individual may find himself. Take, for example, a friend who was finding it difficult to get her two teenage daughters to complete one of their household chores—taking out the garbage. Her strategy had been to discuss with the children the factors that seemed to be inhibiting them from discharging their task. One afternoon a group of us was sitting around giving her advice about how to handle this situation. The consensus was that it was important to discover what was keeping the girls from doing what they were supposed to do. Finally one of the group who had previously been silent asked the woman, "What is it that you want to do?" We all replied as if he were deaf, "Take out the garbage." "Then," he advised firmly, "cut out the discussion and get down to taking out the garbage. It is, after all, what you want done, and apparently they are the ones to do it." We all looked at him dumbstruck. He eyed the woman directly. "Forget the detour of determining why. What you want to do is instill in them the habit of taking out the garbage without being told. After a while it will become routine." Such is the difference between the behavioral and the psychological approach.

Designing and implementing a program of self-management for changing involves the following four elements:

1. Self-knowledge, achieved through self-observation
2. Planning a program and the strategies to implement it
3. Information-gathering and record-keeping on the behavior you wish to change and the progress you make toward meeting your goals
4. Modification of your plans as you proceed in your change

This type of self-management program has been used effectively to modify eating habits among obese patients.[2] In fact, some specialists feel that self-management is the only process that successfully alters dietary patterns in a manner that produces long-term weight loss.[3] In other words, self-management is essential to taking weight off and keeping it off. This is what the experts call *compliance* to a new dietary regimen.

In our food allergy dietary modification program we have

similar goals: it will be necessary for you to induce a change in your eating habits and to be able to maintain that change so that it becomes second nature. Specifically, your goals in this program can be stated as follows:

1. To successfully complete the desensitization period so that you are nonreactive to your cyclical food allergies and can go on to implement the rotary diversified diet
2. To maintain your adherence to the rotary diversified diet.

Essential to your effort will be an understanding of the role your food habits play in your daily life. You can accomplish this by identifying situations and circumstances that may cause you to eat the foods to which you react. In this process you will be describing your regular mealtime patterns, as well as admitting any peculiar habits you might have developed, particularly under pressure or stress. You can then select from a variety of strategies to help you adjust your eating habits to avoid the foods that bother you. These coping strategies are really quite simple:

1. You can learn to manage the cues or antecedents that cause you to eat.
2. You can substitute other activities that make it difficult to indulge in your troublesome behavior. This is what the psychologists call *incompatible behavior.*
3. You can change the consequences or results of your eating patterns.[4]

Each alternative has some specific methods for implementation and can be used singly or in combination, depending on the strength of your negative food habits.

We all have different attitudes about change. One person may engineer a head-on conflict between his present behavior, which has some desirable aspects to it, and the thing he is striving for, which he hopes will be more desirable. Another person may fear change as the difference between the known and comfortable and the unknown and frightening. The experts tell us, however, that the most constructive view is to anticipate change as a chance to implement a harmonious adjustment between yourself and your environment. Humans intuitively strive for harmony in their lives, between their thoughts and emotions, their values and actions, and especially their goals and their capability to achieve them. For a person embarking on a program of self-managed change, the crucial match is between his actions and the situations to which those actions apply. The demands of your environment will affect your behavior, and, conversely, your behavior in one given situation will affect subsequent actions in other similar circumstances.[5]

Harmonious adjustment is not a static goal but rather a continuing process. This is where many of us experience frustration. We establish rigid rules for ourselves to which we attempt religious adherence. In our haste to make these rules, we often tend to underestimate the variety of factors that might influence our ability to stick by them. In this aspect our rules seem to take on the quality of an abstraction, existing without context. Establishing arbitrary rules for behavior without considering the various circumstances to which those rules may apply ultimately results in failure.

This thought relates to the second problem we have when we develop rules. We tend to ignore the necessity of developing backup strategies in case our rules fail us. A rule is a very arbitrary thing, indicating the need for exact compliance in the variety of circumstances to which it might seem applicable. On the other hand, the alternative to rules—guidelines—suggests courses of action that can be molded to meet the needs of a range of situations. Guidelines provide us with a general approach and with the ultimate, most practical tool: the capacity to adjust to circumstances as they happen.

The discovery that you have multiple sclerosis is a case in point. Despite the fact that this was not a change in your life which you desired, it requires adaptation. In this case, adaptation doesn't necessarily mean an arbitrary confrontation with reality, so that you become resigned to your disease. Rather, it means analyzing the circumstances in your life that could be affected by your MS and making the necessary behavior changes to allow you to continue living your life with a minimum of compromise.

By suggesting self-managed behavior as an alternative to the usual coping strategies recommended to MS patients, we are offering guidelines instead of rules. Many people try to "beat" MS by ignoring the ramifications of their disease and attempting to maintain the status quo. Although on good days this might be a feasible strategy, on the inevitable bad ones, when you can't do as much as you'd like, it might cause you unnecessary and unproductive frustration and anxiety. Using self-managed behavior to keep your food allergies in check provides the initial step in constructive adaptation to the realities of living with multiple sclerosis.

Another problem associated with rule-making is that routine adherence depends on that elusive quality, willpower. The word implies a kind of magical quality, perhaps even a matter of luck, as if some people are born with it and others aren't. We tend to applaud the people who appear to have it and are concerned for those who appear to be lacking it. To be precise, what we are born with and can develop are the elements that constitute willpower. These include foresight, the ability to understand cause and effect, and the capacity to plan and develop strategy. Understood this way, willpower is not an elusive abstraction but a skill you can cultivate.

Having constructed an initial statement of your goals—to complete the desensitization period successfully so you can go on to implement the rotary diversified diet and then to successfully maintain an allergy-free state by maintaining adherence to the rotary diet—your next step is to identify those situations that might compromise your achievement of these goals.

Before you attempt that, however, let's think for a minute about what successful completion of the desensitization period means. First, you will have to avoid totally the foods to which you have allergies. This means no slipups, or you'll have to start all over again. It means that you may find yourself feeling sorry for yourself over the foods you have been forced to eliminate from your diet. If the theory runs true, the foods you're going to be giving up for three months are likely to be those you enjoy the most. You could look at it another way, however. You might consider yourself the lucky one. You know what you can't eat, whereas your friend might be suffering from any number of chronic symptoms and have no idea why.

Further on the plus side, completing the desensitization period means you can reintroduce your troublesome foods into your diet. With a little planning, you can eat your favorite foods, from which you've abstained for three months and despaired of ever seeing again. Think what that is to look forward to. The bad news was your discovery of your food allergies. The good news is that now you know which foods cause you trouble, and you have a system that will allow you to eat those foods without experiencing an adverse effect.

Taking first things first, let's start with your goal to complete desensitization successfully. You have already made a list of the foods you must avoid, and you are aware of the various configurations in which they may appear. By this time you should also have made up your list of substitutes and where to find them, which will help you get through this stage. Although your goal is to desensitize yourself to your cyclical allergies, the strategies we are discussing can also be used to help you avoid your fixed allergies. Because those cyclical allergies developed as a result of over exposure to foods, you will be looking for evidence of chronically recurring eating patterns. First and easiest, you will be identifying circumstances that are directly related to eating a particular food—a tendency to grab a piece of chocolate when a certain friend calls for a long chat, the habit of fixing a certain kind of meal under a particular set of circumstances (when you're late or running out of time), or rewarding specific behavior with a favorite food. One writer, for example, allowed himself a bowl of pistachios at the end of a full day of work.

The second factor you must evaluate is the occurrence of an emotional reaction related to your food habits. Do you rationalize an extra cup of coffee and a doughnut as compensation for a bad morning at work? Do you rush to the cookie jar after a hard day? Or is it a glass of wine or a bowl of corn chips? It is important that you evaluate both aspects of the situation—your actual behavior and any emotions that might contribute to that behavior. It won't do you any good to attempt to change your actions if you ignore the emotional overtones that might be affecting it. Research tells us that people often tend to overeat or disrupt their normal eating patterns when they're angry, frustrated, or depressed. Watch out for these circumstances because they're the greatest hidden challenges to your plan for change.

Let's leave the secondary sleuthing until later, however, and concentrate on your eating patterns, especially regarding the foods to which you know you're allergic.

Say, for example, that an individual has discovered that he has an allergy to dairy products. His first step would be to think over the list of dairy products that caused a reaction during his testing and review the occasions on which he tends to eat them. He would have to evaluate all the foods he consumes at each meal, remembering to include snacks. If he looked over his seven most recent breakfasts, for example, he might discover that he's taken to settling for coffee with cream and sugar as a quick way to get started in the morning when he doesn't have time to eat. On the weekends, however, when he has the time for a leisurely breakfast, his preference—like Mr. Bond's—is for bacon, eggs, and toast. He might find that on days when his morning at the office has not gone well he slips out to a small drugstore that makes its own ice cream and downs a vanilla milk shake or a double-dip strawberry cone. On the other hand, when he's feeling OK, he will usually opt for a chef's salad for lunch.

You're looking for a pattern, which may be so ingrained that it might not be obvious. One MS patient, for example, evaluated his hectic round of daily activities as director of development for a small private college and discovered quite to his amazement that he was eating two pounds of raw peanuts a day. His compulsion wasn't born out of emotion or stress but out of the fact that he rarely had time to eat properly, and peanuts were a quick, easy food that provided him with lots of energy. Guess what he ate, however, when he did have time to sit down for a proper lunch—a peanut butter sandwich. Guess what he turned out to be allergic to?

Another individual routinely ate a half gallon of ice cream before he went to bed at night, regardless of what he'd had for dinner. A self-made man who became one of the biggest developers in California, he explained that he ate the ice cream because he "likes the way it tastes." When he thought about it, however, he decided it gave him a feeling of well-being, despite whatever disquieting events might have happened during the day. Further questioning produced the thought that his unusually large consumption of ice cream was a kind of convoluted symbol of success. As a small child growing up in rural Texas, he—among all his friends—rarely had enough money for an ice cream cone.

The pattern you're searching for might be so obvious that you'll miss it, so be careful. When you established the menus for your rotary diet, we encouraged you to take a look at your general patterns—milk and cereal for breakfast or a sandwich at lunch—so you could attempt to duplicate them, at least initially. What you are doing here is investigating such preferences in greater detail. You should allow at least two weeks for this effort. Researchers advise that, if you're working with a typical two-week period, you will probably generate enough data for your observations to be reliable. Such would be true, of course, if your two weeks are typical of your usual schedule. This means that during your two observation weeks there should be no vacations, sicknesses, or other kinds of abnormal situations.

The easiest and most effective strategy for accomplishing your data collection is to use a seven-day calendar, similar to the one you used in planning your rotary diet. Simply enter all the foods you eat each day, being careful to note the quantity. An occasional piece of cake is obviously much less significant than half a cake regularly devoured at one sitting. Be sure to describe any emotions you feel might have contributed to what you ate, be they positive or negative.

Once you have your troublesome food situations identified, you are ready to develop strategies to avoid their temptations. To do this you may use one or all of three coping strategies that will help you change your behavior: (1)

control of the consequences of your behavior; (2) changing the cues that set you off in the first place; and (3) instituting incompatible behavior.

CONSEQUENCES

Let's look at what it might be like to change the consequences of your behavior. Take, for example, the individual who's allergic to dairy products but still continues to soothe his wounded pride with a milk shake after his boss criticizes him unnecessarily. The first thing he would do is identify the consequences of his actions. Before he knew of his allergy to milk his reaction to the shake was probably a feeling of well-being. His boss was angry at him over a trifle, which made him feel inadequate, and indulgence in a favorite food lessened the hurt. To salve his conscience about the milk shake indulgence, he switched to salads for lunch on the uneventful days.

Now that he knows he's allergic to dairy products, the milk shake should not seem to be such a treat since he's aware of its effects. With this in mind, he might be able to avoid the ice cream for a while, until the day the boss really blows up. If he doesn't plan for this kind of situation, he might not be able to cope and will end up cheating.

However, if he developed an alternative outcome for this situation, then the chances are much better that he would be able to avoid his standard reaction. What if he established a reward for himself? Let's say he develops a point system: every time he resists the urge to have ice cream or any kind of dairy product, he gives himself one point and saves his points toward something special he'd like, maybe a new set of golf clubs. Perhaps one point equals one dollar. You can calculate the number of situations in which he would have to be successful before he could plunk down the money for the clubs. Or, if this seems too excessive, he could make a deal with himself that his goal is to accumulate points equal to half the cost of the clubs he wants to buy, to which he will add the other half out of his pocket. This is called *self-reward* or *self-enforcement*. Very simply stated, it means that you determine the behavior you want to exchange for your current undesirable behavior, and then you reward yourself for completing that new behavior.

The keys to successfully implementing a change in the consequences of your behavior are to select for your reinforcement something that you really want and might not ordinarily get and then to establish a reasonable system that makes it possible for you to obtain it. If you feel that your undesirable behavior is very ingrained (valuable to you), establish a punishment that provides a threat to keep you in line. Finally, if you feel the least bit intimidated, enlist the aid of a friend to help you with your self-monitoring and administering your reward. Obviously either you or your friend has to keep records. The simpler, the better. A weekly calendar marked with the times you were tempted and persevered would do it, just as long as it's something that you can use to add up your score.

If you think you have a real problem on your hands, then you might also want to develop a strategy to punish yourself if you slip. Perhaps for our sensitive friend, milk shakes are only the tip of the iceberg, overshadowing Roquefort cheese, his mother's homemade yogurt, and baked goods loaded with milk, butter, and cream. To give himself a better chance he could dock himself $2 every time he slips. This would mean that a slip would cost him twice as much as he would earn by complying with his new behavior. Don't forget that to accomplish your system of monetary rewards and losses, you'll have to keep written records and be conscientious about it.

Although we know self-punishment can be effective, it is not wise to implement a system based solely on punishment. Research tells us that a self-management plan based entirely on self-punishment is not nearly as effective as one that uses self-reinforcement or a combination of both.[6] Your goal, after all, is to make the new behavior second nature, and it won't be unless you practice it. A system using both reward and punishment is effective because it is obvious that unless you make a concerted effort to perform the desired behavior you will end up taking one step forward and two steps back.

During the three-month desensitization period, however, you can't afford any slips, or you'll have to start all over again. The experts say that in this kind of situation the key is to plan a punishment so severe that it will never be implemented— just the threat is enough to keep you on the straight and narrow. Theoretically, the threat of having to start the desensitization period all over again should be enough. If it's not, you should definitely plan some form of self-punishment. If you own something that is very precious—for example, a collection of glassware or a carefully tended herb garden—you might instruct your accomplice that, if you falter, he or she is to destroy something from that collection. And then don't falter.

In implementing your self-managed change, the experts advise that, above all, you must ignore the inevitable urge you will have to cheat. Most people give in to the urge to indulge in something "they are not supposed" to have because they feel that the urge will increase in intensity to the point that it becomes irresistible. Research shows, however, that if you ignore their initial appearance, such urges will gradually subside.[7] They recommend that you prepare a speech to yourself for such occasions; something like, "I will feel better if I don't eat (or drink) that. This urge will not get worse, it will actually go away if I ignore it. Giving in is not worth the trouble it will cause and will only make the urge worse the next time."

Remember that it may also be helpful to have someone assist you in your plan of self-reinforcement. You could get a good friend to hold the reward money. Reporting to someone else on your progress can often be very helpful, especially in the beginning. An assistant to help you monitor your progress is not a bad idea either. Not only is it more difficult to cheat if you have to report to someone on your actions, it's also nice to know that somebody's rooting for you and cares about your struggle.

CUES

To give yourself a head start you could implement the second strategy you have available: you could adjust the cues that lead you to your undesirable behavior. Let's take the case of the young woman who discovers that on nights when she's at home alone she's developed the habit of eating a grilled cheese sandwich for dinner. She developed the habit from those nights she worked as a volunteer in a senior citizens center. She no longer works at the center but finds that she has taken to shopping in the evening and running small errands, and this makes her late. Unfortunately, this woman is allergic to gluten and shouldn't be eating bread.

She has a number of options for changing the cues that deliver her to her grilled cheese sandwich. First she could rearrange her schedule. She could come home for dinner before doing her errands, so she's not as hungry and tired and can fix a meal. Or she could arrange to eat dinner in a restaurant on the nights she does her errands, or do her errand shopping with a friend and invite her home for dinner—hopefully, her sense of hospitality would ensure that she doesn't serve grilled cheese sandwiches, however late they arrive home.

The individual who uses milk shakes to soothe his bruised ego might select another place to eat his lunch, preferably one that doesn't serve milk shakes, perhaps a health food restaurant. If he were having a particularly difficult time resisting the urge, he might go sit in a park for fifteen minutes before he decides on a place to eat. Another alternative is to eliminate the emotional cues that lead to the undesirable behavior. One commonly used method is a quick meditation to slow down breathing and calm the emotions. There are many books available on meditation. If you've just started, you might want to try a guided meditation that gives you instructions on how to clear your mind as part of the meditation exercise itself. You could also engage in some other kind of quieting activity. Take your sewing or your chessboard to the office and have it on hand in case. Find a quiet place and darn a sock or practice a few chess moves.

Another cue change strategy is to break the chain of events that rumble inevitably toward the undesirable behavior. Often it's not one cue, but a series, which causes the troublesome behavior. Our man with the dairy allergy might want to put an end to the situation in which his boss dresses him down. He could sit down and explain to his manager that he can't continue to work that way. If he won't cooperate, his next step might be to discuss the matter with his boss's superior. If that doesn't work, he might seriously consider changing jobs. Anyway, the milk shakes are only a cover-up for a problem he should have confronted in the first place.

The nice thing about taking the time to change the cues that initiate the chain of events leading to bad behavior is that it makes it that much easier for you to collect your reward. Each time your cue change rewards you by inhibiting the behavior you want to avoid, then you can add another installment to your reward fund.

Incompatible Behavior

If you are still having problems, you might try the third strategy. This requires the institution of some kind of incompatible behavior, which makes it impossible to do whatever it is that you want to avoid. But there is one important essential you must include: planning. You must develop your scheme of incompatible behavior beforehand, or you'll discover yourself in a tempting situation armed with nothing but that flimsy willpower. Our dairy addict could join a gym, for example, and schedule his visits during lunch. Better yet, he could make arrangements with a friend to work out together. Not only would he avoid his shakes, but he might lose weight in the process, which could provide an additional incentive. He could also prepare his lunch and take it to work, making sure that he doesn't have enough money to buy lunch and telling his friends what he's doing so they won't let him borrow money if he asks. The young woman with the grilled cheese sandwich problem could engage in the most incompatible behavior of all—not buying bread, so she couldn't make a sandwich even if she wanted one, unless she made a special trip to the store. By then, she could have cooked the chicken breast lying conspicuously in the fridge or bought a roast chicken.

The secret is to acknowledge the danger signs. Know what situations can cause you to trip up and plan for them. Figure out what you're going to do so that when you're faced with temptation you can fall back on a strategy instead of floundering around, anxious and defenseless. An additional recommendation is to practice your new behavior. Thus, the individual who is going to confront his boss would go through the full scenario—his boss shouts, he becomes upset, his stomach starts to turn, and he says to himself, "What I need to calm me down is a vanilla shake. I can't wait 'till noon." That completed, he would now substitute his new scene: "I'm angry, my boss did it to me again; as soon as the bell rings, I'm going to put on my running shoes and go for a fast walk in the park." You can practice verbally, which is the best way, or you can run through it in your mind.

If you are stumped about just how to handle the situation, you might want to model your behavior on someone else. Select someone who is operating in a situation similar to yours and observe how he handles it. Do this on three or four occasions or for however long it takes for you to understand what's happening and how to imitate it. You don't necessarily have to do this from behind a potted palm tree, however. In fact, you might want to approach the person, tell him what you're doing, that you admire how he handles himself and would like to observe how he does it. This might work well for the man who is having troubles with his boss. The first strategy is called rehearsing and the second, modeling. Both are worth taking the time to learn and implement.

This brings us to another guideline. If you feel yourself overwhelmed by all of this, take two steps back and look at yourself and your problem from the perspective of an outsider. First, consider the advantages of not changing. In this case not changing would mean that you get to eat what you want, whenever you want it. This will mean that you may have a sense of well-being—of feeling full or satisfied, whatever the feeling is that you reserve for your favorite foods. Eating the food might take your mind off something that's bothering you; it might brighten your day to go on a spree, especially if you've been feeling sorry for yourself. You might also want to argue in the name of practicality, i.e., you don't have the time to bother with all of this. All of which might be true, but you are still left with the problems that suggested change in the first place: a reaction to foods that causes you to have unpleasant symptoms and aggravates your MS.

Researchers tell us that one of the reasons people have trouble changing is that they haven't thought through what the change will entail.[8] Thus, when they're confronted with a tempting situation, they say to themselves, "I didn't know that giving up such and such was going to mean that." If the young woman with the grilled cheese sandwiches thought it out and realized that it would take her longer to cook a chicken breast than to quick fry a sandwich, she could prepare herself. Perhaps she could cook the chicken on Sunday and freeze it or get home an hour earlier. But if she doesn't plan adequately, and then arrives home at her usually late hour and opens the fridge to an admittedly unappetizing pink chicken, she is just leaving herself open to the temptation of pulling out the frying pan and melting the cheese. At that point she has no options. Your options are open only *before* you find yourself in your difficult situation. Then, you can plan.

After you have evaluated the reasons that might inhibit your making your prospective change you should consider the benefits of making the change. Your health is obviously one. There is also the fact that when you get through this period you will be able to eat your formerly troublesome foods without awakening the symptoms of food allergy and your MS. You will also have the satisfaction of doing something about your disease, instead of fearing the future in a wheelchair.

Generally speaking, in dealing with consummatory behaviors such as overeating or drug or alcohol addiction, you're better off concerning yourself with short-term gains than long-term goals.[9] So don't spend time with the thought that this program will keep you mobile and self-sufficient five years from now; think instead that tomorrow you'll be able to walk, talk and generally carry on your life as you'd like. Researchers and therapists also have found that people with weight problems tend to concentrate on the times when they fall off their diet, often indulging in serious self-criticism while forgetting to congratulate themselves when they succeed.[10] You should make it a rule to use your self-monitoring information as an opportunity to congratulate yourself as you progress. If you come very close to giving in to your food urge, think of all the times you didn't. If you do slip, however, stop yourself immediately, pat yourself on the back for all the good work you've done, and get back to business. Don't, by any means, start to feel sorry for yourself or berate yourself for slipping up, because then you run the risk of using your failure as an excuse to continue your mistake and indulge in a big way. If you criticize yourself unmercifully for a mistake, you can fall into the rationalization of "Well, as long as I'm at it, I might as well make it a whopper." That's giving your slip far too much power. Just pass it by and get back on track.

After you've considered the pluses and minuses of your proposed change in behavior, and hopefully opted for the pluses, you should spend some time evaluating your ability to change. If you've done all the things you should have— established goals, observed your present behavior, and developed your strategies, including a system whereby you can monitor your progress—then you should have little trouble with your campaign. Your proposed change will happen, and you should believe it. If you look at your preparations and sit around and fret about whether or not you can pull this off, chances are you won't. You'll end up in the heap with the people who say that the effort is too much, life is too short, and they're happier with their shakes and grilled cheese sandwiches.

There are various estimates of how long it takes to change a habit—anywhere from three weeks to many months—but there appears to be general agreement that you will want to do it slowly, with a multifaceted approach, not with an impatient, head-on confrontation. It took you awhile to develop your habit patterns, so it will take you awhile to change them. Gradually you'll get to the point where you forget to give yourself your reinforcement and your behavior will constitute its own reward. After you reach that goal, it would not be a bad idea to drop back into your reward system once in a while.

Research seems to indicate that intermittent reinforcement works better than cutting off the reinforcement system completely.[11] You may want to change your system a bit. You might have reached the stage where you're performing the new behavior and as a consequence are enjoying your new golf clubs. Now perhaps you should start saving for a new bag or a pair of shoes. Or maybe you'd prefer adding one dollar to the kitty for every week you stay on target and put that away to buy something special for yourself or someone else. You would not do it every week, but perhaps every other week, or on no schedule at all. Intermittent reinforcement of this type, however, recalls your attention to your plan and your ability to maintain it. This makes you stop a minute and gives you a chance to feel good about yourself.

And you should feel good. You did it. You made it through the three months, and you're ready to proceed with the diet you've planned.

10

ESSENTIAL STRATEGIES FOR DISCOVERING YOUR ALLERGIES AND DEVELOPING A DIET

This is the refrigerator chapter. What you do is take these pages, cut them out, and put them on your refrigerator door. Then you won't have any excuses. In this chapter you've got the whole thing from start to finish, down in black and white, so all you have to do is look. No excuses: "I couldn't find the book," "My son took it to school," or "The maid threw it out."

The first thing you do from here, before you even finish reading the rest of the book, is take these pages and cut them out. Then put them up on the refrigerator with those little magnets you buy in the supermarket or tack them on the wall somewhere where you will see them. Do you have a desk where you do your work? Tape them up over your desk. Do you do your menu planning in the kitchen? Then buy a bulletin board and pin them on it. Do whatever it takes to get this material in front of you so you'll use it.

We want you to use it; that's why we wrote the book. So here we go, from the beginning.

THE SIX QUESTIONS

1. What foods are you sure you're not allergic to?

2. What foods do you suspect you are allergic to?
3. What foods do you eat at least once a day?
4. Which foods would it be the most difficult to give up?
5. Which foods could you easily replace?
6. What are your favorite foods?

Cross off the answers to numbers 2 and 5. These are probably your safe foods. Make a list of all the foods you identified in answering the other four questions—1, 3, 4, and 6. This is **List A.** Use it for the pulse and niacin tests.

THE PULSE AND NIACIN TESTS

1. Eat your regular meals for three days.
2. Take your pulse before you get up in the morning, before each meal, and 30, 60, and 90 minutes after each meal. Check your pulse once more at bedtime. Take the niacin, 100 milligrams, an hour before eating and watch for flushing 5–30 minutes after eating. Use a watch with a second hand. Count your pulse each time for a full minute. Avoid snacks; include them in your meal.
3. List all the foods you had at the meals that caused your pulse to rise at least 16 beats over your pre-rising rate (or 6 beats over your pre-meal rate). This is **List B.** You will use it for your mini-meal test.

THE MINI-MEAL TEST

1. Gather together all the foods that caused your pulse to rise; set aside three or four days; make yourself six mini-meals each day using only one each of the foods for each meal—a glass of milk, a piece of bread, etc. Allow three hours for each food. Take your pulse before each "meal" and at 30, 60, and 90 minutes afterward. Take your niacin the same way you did during the initial pulse and niacin testing. If your pulse has not returned to within three-four beats of the pre-meal rate, delay the next mini-meal test for an additional hour.
2. Make a list of all the foods that cause a reaction. This is

List C. These are the foods you will be testing in the rotary diversified diet. Sustain yourself during this period on your safe foods, which you know don't cause a reaction. Test one of the reactive foods each day or every other day until you've tested all the foods on List C.

THE ROTARY DIVERSIFIED DIET

1. Initially, abstain from all the food on List C and eat only your safe foods. Continue to take your pulse and niacin tests as before.
2. After several days of safe foods, start at the top of List C and reintroduce the first food at one meal. Observe and describe any symptoms.
3. After one or two days, reintroduce the second food on the list, again at only one meal; complete the pulse and niacin tests and observe symptoms.
4. Continue down the list until you've tested all the foods in the same manner. Each time you eat a new food, observe and note your symptoms along with your test results. This is very important. If you experience any dramatic symptoms, wait for all the symptoms to clear before you attempt to test another food.
5. Stop when you get to the bottom of the list; if you have any foods that didn't cause a reaction when you went back on them, cross them off the list, at least for now. The remaining foods on List C are your primary food allergens. Put your reaction on the page next to the food. You now have **List D**.

THE DESENSITIZATION PERIOD

1. Sit down and recap your regular eating patterns for the last two weeks. List all the foods you ate at each meal, including snacks.
2. Try to remember whether you are aware of any emotional reaction before, during, or after eating. Include

your description of your feelings with your description of your meal. You should continue to do this throughout your desensitization period.
3. Plan how you're going to break the patterns: reward yourself for good behavior, change the cues that cause you to eat; use incompatible behavior.
4. Using List D, the foods you have to avoid, you will need to develop at least one week's worth of menus which you can rotate throughout the three-month desensitization period.
5. Obtain foods and other supplies.
6. Stay with it.

DEVELOPING THE ROTARY DIET

1. Maintain four days between individual foods, two days between families.
2. Eat only fresh, unprocessed food; cook it simply.
3. Check all ingredients; don't guess.
4. Don't cheat.
5. Don't start until you're desensitized; remember, it takes three months.
6. Plan menus carefully; keep records of your menus.

THE FOOD GROUPS

1. Check the food groups; list all the foods you know and like.
2. List all the foods you would like to try.
3. If you don't know where to buy the unusual foods, scout out the sources. Next to each food, write down where you can buy it.
4. Get whatever other supplies you need—nonstick pans, cookbooks, etc.
5. Decide if you want to use food substitutes; if you do, find out where to buy them.
6. After you try a new food, make a note of how you liked it.

For your convenience, here is a listing of food groups and food families within each group.

PLANT

Fruits

Apple—apple, pear, quince
Banana—banana, plantain
Citrus—citron, grapefruit, kumquat, lemon, lime, orange, tangerine
Gooseberry—currant, gooseberry
Heather—blueberry, cranberry, huckleberry, wintergreen
Mulberry—fig, hop, mulberry
Palm—coconut, date, sago
Plum—almond, apricot, cherry, nectarine, peach, plum (prune)
Rose—blackberry, boysenberry, dewberry, loganberry, raspberry, strawberry,
chestnut, elderberry, grape (raisins), litchi nut, papaya, pineapple, pomegranate

Vegetables

Beet—beet, chard, lambs-quarters, spinach
Buckwheat—buckwheat, rhubarb
Composite—artichoke, chicory, dandelion, endive, escarole, Jerusalem artichoke, lettuce, salsify, sunflower
Fungus—mushroom, yeast
Ginger—ginger, turmeric
Laurel—avocado, bay leaf, cinnamon, sassafras
Legume—beans, carob, cowpea, lentil, licorice, pea, peanut, soybean, tragacanth gum
Lily—asparagus, chive, garlic, leek, onion
Mallow—cottonseed, okra
Mustard—broccoli, Brussels sprout, cabbage, celery cabbage, cauliflower, collard, horseradish, kale, mustard, mustard greens, radish, rutabaga, turnip, watercress

Parsley—anise, caraway, carrot, celery, coriander, dill, fennel, parsley, parsnip

Potato—cayenne, chili, eggplant, green pepper, paprika, potato, red pepper, tobacco, tomato

Walnut—butternut, hickory nut, pecan, walnut

arrowroot, filbert (hazelnut) ginseng, macadamia nut, maple, olive, pine nut, sesame, sweet potato, tapioca, taro, vanilla, water chestnut

Mixed Fruits and Vegetables

Cashew—cashew, mango, pistachio

Gourd—cantaloupe, cucumber, melons, pumpkin, squashes

Grain

Cereal—bamboo, barley, corn, millet, oat, rice, rye, sorghum, sugar cane, triticale, wheat, wild rice

Herbs, Spices, and Flavorings

Mint—basil, horehound, marjoram, mint, oregano, peppermint, sage, savory, spearmint, thyme

Nutmeg—nutmeg, mace

Pepper—black and white

Sterculia—chocolate, cocoa, cola

Vanilla

Miscellaneous

Coffee

Tea

ANIMAL

Birds

1. *Chicken, pheasant, quail*
2. *Duck, goose*
3. *Grouse*

4. *Guinea hen*
5. *Turkey*

Eggs of the birds are considered to be of the same family as the parent bird.

Fish

Ocean
Cod—cod (scrod), haddock, hake
Croaker—croaker, drum, sea trout, silver perch, weakfish
Decapods—crab, crayfish, lobster, prawn, shrimp
Flounder—flounder, halibut, plaice, sole, turbot
Herring—menhaden, sardine, sea herring, shad
Mackerel—albacore, bonito, mackerel, skipjack, tuna
Pelecypods—clam, mussel, oyster, scallop
Sea Bass—grouper, sea bass, red snapper
Fresh water
Catfish—bullhead, catfish
Perch—sauger, walleye, yellow perch
Pike—pickerel, northern pike, muskellunge
Salmon—salmon species, trout species
Sunfish—black bass species, bluegill, crappy, sunfish
Single Families
Abalone; Anchovy; Bluefish; Carp; Eel; Lake Whitefish; Mullet; Ocean Catfish; Ocean Perch; Shark; Smelt; Squid; Sturgeon; Swordfish; Tilefish; Ocean Whitefish

Mammals

1. **Bovines**—bison, buffalo, cattle, goats, sheep.
2. **Caribou, deer, elk, moose.**
3. **All other mammals commonly eaten, including rabbit, squirrel, and swine.**

A SAMPLE CASE

To demonstrate how the system works, let's review a typical case. We suggest that you pay special attention to the format used to collect the data. Blanks of these forms are provided in the appendix.

When we applied the six questions to this case, we obtained the following answers.

1. Foods the individual feels he is most likely not allergic to: milk, beef, oranges, tomatoes, wheat
2. Foods he most suspects: eggs, chicken/turkey, green beans, cucumbers
3. Foods he eats once a day or more: milk, bread, or some kind of cereal-type product, oranges or orange juice, potatoes.
4. The most difficult foods for him to give up: ice cream, yogurt, milk, potatoes, coffee, bread, cake and other baked goods, beef (especially steaks and hamburgers), chocolate
5. The easiest things for him to give up: fish, vegetables (except tomatoes and lettuce)
6. His favorite foods: bread, hamburgers, milk, ice cream, chocolate, steak, orange juice, french fries

From these answers, **List A** was formulated:

List A

milk	bread
oranges	cake
tomatoes	chocolate
potatoes	hamburgers
ice cream	steak
yogurt	

After a four-day fast the three-day pulse test and niacin tests were initiated. Figure 1 shows what the meals looked like, along with the pulse and flushing reactions to each meal. Notice that we implemented the nonsnack recommendation. The chocolate cake and the cookies ordinarily would have been eaten as snacks, but for purposes of the test we included them in the preceding meals.

FIGURE 1—Pulse & Niacin Tests (Regular Diet)

FOODS EATEN	PULSE	NIACIN
Day One	Pre-Rising *61*	**REACTION**

BREAKFAST

orange juice, plain	Premeal *64*	
wheat, milk, black	30 min. *80 (+19)*	*yes*
coffee	60 min. *75*	
	90 min. *68*	

LUNCH

tuna sandwich with	Premeal *65*	
lettuce and tomato, iced	30 min. *67*	
tea	60 min. *72*	*yes*
	90 min. *69*	

DINNER

hamburger on bun,	Premeal *66*	
french fries, lettuce, tomato,	30 min. *74*	
ketchup, milk, chocolate	60 min. *83 (+22)*	*yes*
brownie	90 min. *75*	

Day Two	Pre-Rising *64*	

BREAKFAST

orange juice, cottage	Premeal *67*	
cheese, bran muffin,	30 min. *74*	
butter, black coffee	60 min. *81 (+17)*	*yes*
	90 min. *71*	

LUNCH

sliced turkey sandwich	Premeal *68*	
with mustard, rice	30 min. *70*	
cake, milk	60 min. *75*	*yes*
	90 min. *67*	

DINNER

steak, salad with	Premeal *68*	
lettuce, tomato, and	30 min. *84 (+20)*	
cucumber, mashed potatoes,	60 min. *78*	*yes*
chocolate cake, milk	90 min. *72*	

Figure 1 (continued)

Day Three   Pre-Rising *65*

BREAKFAST

tomato juice, scrambled   Premeal *68*
eggs, toast, butter,   30 min. *85 (+20)* *yes*
white grapes, black   60 min. *78*
coffee   90 min. *73*

LUNCH

vanilla milk shake   Premeal *69*
chocolate chip cookies   30 min. *80*
                                 60 min. *83 (+18)* *yes*
                                 90 min. *70*

DINNER

swordfish with lemon, boiled   Premeal *70*
potatoes, green beans,   30 min. *72*
orange juice, lettuce   60 min. *73*   *no*
and tomato salad   90 min. *66*

From the the results of the pulse and niacin tests, **List B** was developed. This list was used for the mini-meal test.

List B

milk	rice cake
yogurt	tuna
butter	turkey
ice cream	eggs
cottage cheese	black coffee
chocolate chip cookies	tea
chocolate fudge	mustard
oranges	cane sugar
steak	vinegar and oil
white bread	almonds
bran muffin	

You can see by the ingredients that we added at the end that it is not always easy to remember to record everything.

Sometimes what you eat is so routine that you forget about it. This is why you should work with your physician or some other knowledgeable person as you complete these tests. You need someone who will prod your memory.

If you study Figure 1, you'll notice that the pre-rising pulse rate is exceeded by more than 16 beats on DAY ONE. This happens twice on DAY TWO, and twice on DAY THREE. In each of these meals, either coffee or a food containing chocolate was eaten. These were not the only problems, however. Potential difficulties with other foods are still indicated because the pulse rate rose more than six beats per minute above the pre-meal rate after all the other meals, except for dinner on DAY THREE. The results for this meal probably indicate that the foods eaten were well tolerated by this individual and thus probably didn't add significantly to the reactions recorded for the other meals. At this stage, our records indicate that this person's maximum daily resting pulse rate would appear to be either 73 or 75, depending on how much importance we ascribe to the flushing of the niacin reaction. In these tests, because there was a variety of food at each meal, it was difficult to accurately ascribe the flushing to a particular food or type of food. The subsequent mini-meal test, however, helped determine more precisely what foods were actually contributing to the niacin flush.

Figure 2 shows the results of the mini-meal test. You'll notice that several foods that were on List B again showed significant reactions in this test, specifically all milk products, chocolate, wheat, eggs, coffee, and tea. You'll also notice that we added several items to the list that were not independently evident in the original meals. Sugar and corn syrup are ingredients in many of the foods eaten in eight of the mini-meals. They appeared in the baked goods, the ketchup, the fudge, the ice cream and milk shake, and probably in the French fries, in the form of dextrose which is usually derived from corn. Since most commercial bread contains corn syrup, and corn syrup by itself caused a significant increase in the pulse, as well as a niacin reaction, we can conclude that it was the corn in the bread rather than just the wheat itself that contributed to the resulting reaction. Another food

FIGURE 2—Mini-Meal Tests
(PRE-RISING PULSE 60)

FOOD	PULSE				NIACIN
	Premeal	*30*	*60*	*90*	**REACTION**
milk, ½ glass	64	78	75	72	yes
yogurt, ½ carton	63	79	70	66	yes
butter, 1 tsp.	62	66	74	72	yes
ice cream, ½ cup	64	80	77	70	yes
cottage cheese, ½ cup	65	76	73	70	yes
chocolate chip cookies, 3	63	76	82	74	yes
chocolate fudge, 1 pc.	67	78	84	73	yes
orange ½ medium	68	72	74	67	no
steak 1 med. pc.	67	72	72	70	no
white bread, 1 slice	73	79	80	67	yes
buck wheat ½ cup	63	66	67	66	no
bran muffin	65	78	72	72	yes
rice cake	65	66	65	63	no
wheat cereal (plain), ½ cup	67	76	72	71	yes
tuna	64	66	63	62	no
turkey	62	67	66	63	no
egg, 1 boiled	62	78	80	65	yes
black coffee, ½ cup	64	76	80	65	yes
tea, ½ cup	65	79	76	66	yes
mustard, ¼ tsp.	60	63	65	65	no
white grapes, 6	63	63	65	62	no
corn syrup 1 tsp.	66	76	77	70	yes
cane sugar, 1 tsp. in water	63	70	69	66	no
vinegar tsp.	63	63	63	62	no
oil, 1 tsp.	63	70	67	67	no
almonds, ¼ cup	64	65	61	62	no

found throughout the mini-meals was egg, which is usually contained in ice cream, bran muffins, cake, and mayonnaise.

Because the reactions to cane sugar and oil weren't as significant as the other reactions, these foods were considered to be only possibly allergenic. They were not eliminated from consideration completely, however, but were reserved for testing at another time, after the stronger, more reactive foods were tested.

It's important to remember and understand that if we hadn't isolated several of these items to be tested specifically in the mini-meal test, we wouldn't have been able to determine which of the foods in a combined food product caused the reaction—whether, for example, it was the wheat or corn syrup in the ice cream. You can determine which foods should be tested in this individual way by very carefully checking the ingredients on labels or talking with the person who prepared the food if you weren't the cook.

By the way, for the three days of the pulse test and niacin tests it is advisable not to eat out in a restaurant or at a friend's home. You may have difficulty in determining the ingredients of all the foods you eat. For example, this case included butter; if you were eating in a restaurant, it might be difficult to assess whether butter or margarine was used, as well as the ingredients in the margarine (was corn or safflower oil used as a base?).

From this data we developed **List C,** the foods that would be tested with the rotary diversified diet.

List C

milk	corn syrup
yogurt	corn sugar
butter	corn meal
ice cream	corn scratch
cottage cheese	cakes, cereal or anything
coffee	with wheat flour in it,
tea	including baked goods,
buckwheat	gravies, and sauces
chocolate	

As structured, this is a monthlong test. We also included wheat cereal in the test so we could get a clear reading on the wheat factor. Regarding the reaction to bread, it was possible that the individual was reacting to the yeast as well as the wheat itself, or possibly to the corn sweetener. The fact that there was a reaction to wheat cereal (and to corn syrup) eliminated yeast as a suspect and confirmed the others. We included buckwheat for a similar reason—we wanted to check that the allergic reaction was actually to wheat and not to one of its components, gluten. Buckwheat, you'll remember, is not in the cereal family, but it does contain gluten. Since the individual assured us that these meals were typical of the food he generally ate, we did not include any other foods in the rotary diet test, although it is wise to test any food you eat regularly, regardless of whether or not it appears in the three-day pulse and niacin tests.

Our final list, **List D,** was then formulated—the initial list of troublesome foods. This is the starting point for the dietary modification program and was used to develop menus for the desensitization period.

List D

all dairy products—milk, cream, butter, ice cream, yogurt,
    and all cheeses
corn products—corn sweeteners, corn starch, corn meal,
    dextrose, glucose, etc.
caffeine, including coffee, tea, soft drinks, and other
    caffeine-containing beverages or substances, including
    health medications
bananas
wheat

Figure 3 demonstrates a week's worth of menus that were developed to avoid the defined allergies during the three months of the desensitization period. Although this plan presents one week's menus, at the end of the week, the individual would have a choice—starting again at day one exactly as laid out here or rotating. He could start with day seven, instead of day one. Or start the first week with day one, say Monday, and the next week, with day two, Tuesday. Whichever system is chosen, it's recommended that you plan for a minimum of a week. If you usually shop every two weeks, then plan a two-week menu. The whole point of the exercise is, however, to plan. You must have the food in the house so it's available when you need it.

You'll notice that, in developing our menu, we included some of the foods in the original diet, as well as introducing some new ones. The foods included here are such that they can be purchased in a number of ways. The salmon can be fresh or frozen but not canned. If it's canned, the oil might throw your rotation off. Likewise in any case that calls for margarine, you'd have to check which kind of oil it was made from. If you are allergic to corn, then you'd have to buy safflower margarine. The lobster can be fresh or frozen; the strawberries can be fresh or frozen, depending on the time of the year. It's best to buy them unsweetened if you react to cane sugar or corn sugar. The fact that you react to these substances doesn't mean that you're allergic to the sugar itself, but to the cane or corn contaminants contained in the sugar. You can buy fresh artichokes or frozen ones, as long as they have no sauces or flavors added. Supermarkets now carry corn and rice cereals, and many have no preservatives. You should use those whenever possible. Use brown rice for variety. It has a nutty flavor that tastes good for breakfast. It used to be available only in health food stores, but most markets now carry it. In dishes where you might use flour as a binding—the chicken croquettes, for example—you could use buckwheat or potato or rice flour. Rye crackers come free of wheat flour, but you have to check. Rye bread doesn't, but occasionally you can find a store that carries rice flour bread.

You might want to experiment with using other flours in your baking. But again, don't become compulsive and overdo. Try to keep variety in your diet. Consider the desensitizing period as practice for the opportunities of the rotary diet. Don't buy prepared mixes such as buckwheat pancake mix because it will often contain wheat as well as buckwheat

FIGURE 3—New Diet

DAY ONE

Breakfast

apple juice
rice cereal with almond milk
coffee substitute

Lunch

sliced turkey with rye crackers
cucumber-onion salad with vinegar dill
dressing; sliced pear
fresh orange juice

Dinner

broiled trout with garlic and leeks
boiled potatoes
steamed broccoli with toasted sesame
seeds; watermelon; camomile tea

DAY TWO

Breakfast

cantaloupe
scrambled eggs cooked in non-stick pan
rice bread toast with honey
orange spice tea

Lunch

tuna chunks with Mexican salsa
sliced apple with cinnamon
mineral water

Dinner

poached chicken with mushrooms and
herbs; steamed rice
cold artichoke with vinegar and
peanut oil dip; almond tea

FIGURE 3—New Diet (continued)

DAY THREE

Breakfast

fresh orange juice
buck wheat pancakes with pure
maple syrup; coffee substitute

Lunch

salmon, celery and radish salad
with walnut oil dressing
toasted rice bread; grapes
peppermint tea

Dinner

stir fried chicken with water chest-
nuts and chinese pea pods; rice
poached pear with vanilla and
honey; mineral water

DAY FOUR

Breakfast

steamed brown rice with raisins
and pure maple syrup
almond milk
apple spice tea

Lunch

sliced ham
German potato salad
poached oranges with shredded
coconut; mineral water

Dinner

chicken croquettes made with
rice flour; baked butternut squash
with nutmeg and chicken broth; stewed
prunes and figs; camomile tea

FIGURE 3—New Diet (continued)

DAY FIVE

Breakfast

baked apples
rice cereal with almond or soy milk
coffee substitute

Lunch

avocado stuffed with shrimp salad
with egg dressing; rye crackers
plums
iced mint tea

Dinner

hamburgers with mustard
rice and mushroom pilaf
hearts of lettuce with tomato juice
dressing; fresh or frozen strawberries
camomille tea

DAY SIX

Breakfast

fresh orange juice
buck wheat pancakes with strawberries
coffee substitute

Lunch

salmon patties
cucumber, carrots, and celery spears
with egg dressing dip
watermelon; mineral water

Dinner

lamb chops; potato pancakes
green beans with almonds
peaches with raspberry sauce
peppermint tea

DAY SEVEN   **FIGURE 3—New Diet (continued)**

Breakfast

cantaloupe
poached eggs
coffee substitute

Lunch

lobster salad with pimentos and
green peppers; walnut dressing; rice
crackers grape fruit half with
pure maple syrup; almond tea

Dinner

fried brown rice with onions,
bean sprouts, and chicken
mixed fruit cup
mineral water

flour. If you're allergic to corn, make sure your maple syrup is pure and doesn't contain corn syrup.

Health food stores usually carry coffee substitutes and herb teas, although grocery stores often carry them also, sometimes in the health or gourmet food section. Decaffeinated coffee in not an acceptable substitute for coffee, because virtually all decaffeinated coffees contain a small residue of caffeine.

In addition to carefully selecting the foods in your menus each day, you should avoid large servings of any one food. It is possible that an extremely small quantity of an allergic food or beverage could cause a problem for you. By following this general principle, however, you can minimize an adverse reaction if an allergy or intolerance does exist.

You will also notice that, although this plan tries to make use of leftovers, it also prevents you from using the same food often, so you can minimize the possibility of developing additional cyclical allergies. A final ploy is the addition of flavorings that were totally missing from the original diet, in which salt, sugar, mustard, and tomato were the primary flavorings. One important aspect of this menu which you should notice: the dishes don't require elaborate preparation. You will also notice they don't use prepared foods. "Convenience" foods aren't convenient if they make you sick.

If you feel you can't break the prepared food habit, however, keep these guidelines in mind when you shop:

1. Frozen foods: buy them in the big bag packages rather than in the little boxes. They're more economical; they give you a good supply, so you won't have to worry about having them around when you need them; and they are usually unadulterated by flavorings and additives.

2. Before you buy any frozen food, check how it was prepared. Watch for butter sauces, special flavorings, etc., and for sugar. These aren't good for you and take away from the natural taste of foods.

3. In buying canned foods, you must really watch how the food was prepared. With canned goods, there is much more of a tendency to add ingredients to the cooking process, especially sugar and salt. Some of the major canned-good houses are producing salt- and sugar-free lines. Buy them. If you find you miss the salt or sugar, add some nutmeg or cinnamon to the fruit and garlic or onion powder to the vegetables.

4. In buying flour, read the label to make sure you're getting what you want—pure rye or rice or potato flour, not a mixture. If you're interested in prepared baked goods like muffins or bread or crackers, don't assume that, because the label says rye toast or corn muffins, that's what you're buying. Read the ingredients.

5. Canned fish or meat usually comes packed in oil. Check to see what kind it is; if you're allergic to corn oil and the sardines are swimming in it, don't buy them. Sardines and tuna and other types of canned fish come water-packed. Buy them that way; it eliminates a lot of problems. Avoid buying canned meat. It might contain preservatives and additional flavorings. Buy fresh.

6. Don't get stuck in the rut of using no oil on your salads or margarine on your foods. There are lots of different

kinds of oils on the market that will add more flavor to your food and avoid your allergies. Read the label, however, to make sure it's not a blend. For your general health, however, use it and all oils sparingly.

7. Finally, if you don't see it, ask. Particularly in specialty and health food stores, people are usually knowledgeable and welcome a chance to demonstrate what they know. In these types of establishments people are often familiar with the problems of food allergies. They can help you with substitutes as well as brands and best buys.

In preparing for the three-month desensitization period, we strongly suggest that you equip yourself with a good allergy cookbook. Some of them are very innovative in their approaches, listing recipes by what they don't contain, measurement equivalencies, and unusual substitutes that you might not think of. There's a list in the appendix. Use it; it will make your life much easier.

A few words about eating out. During this time, try to avoid it. You can look forward to it as a treat when you implement your rotary diet; then you can afford a slipup occasionally. During the desensitization stage you can't afford any mistakes, however. If you must eat out, go to a restaurant where you can get something simple—a plain piece of fish or chicken, a simple salad, and vegetables. When you arrive, explain your problem to the waiter. Tell him that when you say plain, you mean it—no butter, *really*. If you know you're going to be tempted by something, make it at home and take it with you: wheat-free muffins, salad dressing, etc. Then don't cheat—eat what you bring with you. Smaller restaurants that specialize in individually prepared foods are probably a better bet than larger institutions that tend to take an assembly line approach.

In all of this you must remember your goal, and you must believe that you can do it. We've talked about self-reinforcement, and we've suggested that you rehearse your actions in situations that you feel might be difficult for you. As you do that, always remember to visualize success. Practicing success is one of the most effective tools you have.

11

OTHER PEOPLE—
YOU NEED THEM, TOO

Scene: The dining room of a prestigious Waterloo restaurant. A big sunny room, decorated in shades of soft gold, accented on this day with pink and white poinsettias. A large western fir is in the center of the room. Hung with antique toys and tiny sparkling lights, it hovers over a huge pile of pink and gold gift boxes.

In summer this room would be filled with golf and tennis partners, along with a few businessmen and an occasional local politician. The rest of the tables would be graced with well-dressed women sipping white wine and eating shrimp salads. The dinners are different at this time of year, however. An office Christmas party crowds the tables at the far end of the large room. There are several other groups of business associates celebrating the end of the year and some local gentry entertaining visiting kin. Table 20 over by the window, however, seems to defy classification. Except that the diners aren't local, they look like three women out for a postshopping lunch. Their voices rise; they seem to be exchanging views with more animation than would befit housewives discussing a new recipe or what to wear on New Year's Eve.

163

Cindy Morse is telling a story about her husband: it had been a cool autumn day in suburban Washington, and she had worked hard. She was polishing the dining room furniture when her husband walked through the door, loaded down with computer manuals. He looked at Cindy as she buzzed around the room finishing her weekly cleaning. *"Come on, kid,"* he said to her. *"Why don't you just sit down? Sit down and rest; you're overdoing."*

Cindy relates how she turned abruptly toward her well-meaning husband and snapped, *"I can't Ron, I'm OK today, and I can't stop."*

The other women laugh and nod knowingly.

Suzanne Baccone asks Cindy if she thinks MS has affected her socially. Cindy answers immediately.

"Oh, yes, I'm more aware of people and what I need from them. I'm also more in touch with what I can give. My parents and Ron's parents have been absolutely terrific. I have always believed that half the battle with MS is that if you have good support, you can make it."

Janet Myerson turns toward Cindy, wagging her finger in Cindy's face to emphasize her words:

"Yes, but one of the most difficult things when you are first diagnosed with MS is that you get no support, none—I don't mean from families—from the people who are supposed to know. You're left on your own. So what do you do? You turn inward. You look to yourself and your family and to your friends, if they're understanding enough. Most of all you pray that the people around you will come through. If not, it can be hell."

Janet continues.

"You have a lot of questions you want to ask someone. You want to yell and scream about what's happening to you, but there's no one to answer your questions. I finally just settled down and said, 'OK, I've got it. Now let's get on with how I deal with it.' Nat was terrific. When I came home from Waterloo I was very weak. I needed help physically. My mind was buzzing right along, though, and I was fearful of someone directing me, telling me what to do. I needed people to understand that I was temporarily out of order and could use a little help until I got better.

"Nat sensed that and gave me enough leeway. We were in sync again, because we had a handle on the problem and were ready to go with it. Like everyone else, we were frustrated and confused at first because we didn't know how to proceed. After Waterloo, however, we had a goal to work for. But you just can't do something like that by yourself. You have to have a partner."

Suzanne's experience was not as easy as Janet's.

"My husband seemed like he didn't care, but that was because he didn't understand. The thing I tell anyone with MS is to get an education. You have to learn as much as you can so you can tell your spouse. Your parents, too, and anyone else close to you. I wanted them all to know that I wasn't going to keel over on them unexpectedly or cause them a lot of horrible problems. But the person you want and need the most from is your spouse. If he's not with you, forget it. I had a real hard time with that. Jack and I almost got divorced."

Suzanne is near tears remembering that time. Cindy reaches over and touches her hand.

"But it has to start with yourself, Suzanne; first you have to understand it, then you can explain it to other people. You have to have knowledge, but you also have to accept that you have the disease and learn to cope with it. I think you were right in going to a therapist. Everyone should get the help they need, then they can help other people help them."

Taking a tissue from Janet, Suzanne wipes her eyes and smiles.

"When I was having all my troubles with Jack I felt like I was going to break apart, so I just did what I had to do. I fell back on my MS friends. They gave me support and advice and a sense of belonging. We exchanged information and experiences, but most of all we helped each other emotionally. You have to know that somebody cares. You need assurance that you're not a freak. It also helps to have someone who will celebrate your progress with you."

Janet explains that her husband's belief that she could and would overcome multiple sclerosis was a crucial factor in her recovery and subsequent adjustment to MS.

"Being brave, that's what it's all about. Being brave and

supportive. His belief that I was going to get better helped immensely. If you can't get strength from the people close to you, it's hard going."

"You know why?" Cindy chimes in. *"Because you get so much other negativity thrown at you. One day, although I was not in very good shape, I wanted to go grocery shopping with my husband. I was in the store and had started loading up the cart. About halfway through I just couldn't stand up any more—probably too much dusting. So Ron got my wheelchair out of the trunk of the car. I try to forget it's there, but he always makes sure we have it, just in case. So he gets the chair out and puts me in it, and I go on about my business. It was in the produce department that this lady got to me. You know how hard it is to get things from the produce section because there's never enough room. But I'm there picking over a batch of potatoes and this woman says to me, 'Watch it, honey; I was here first.' I couldn't believe my ears. Then she says, 'How come you're sitting in that wheelchair anyhow? You look all right to me.'*

"That kind of thoughtlessness just devastates me. It's bad enough that people stare when you're in a wheelchair. They peer at you, trying to figure out what's wrong with you. I hate being thought of as handicapped, but then when they accuse you of cheating, my God."

Janet puts down her fork and grins.

"Your problem, Cindy, is that you're too sensitive about what other people think. Goodness gracious, my dear, what's more important—your health and well-being or some nerd who's stupid and impolite?"

Cindy looks over at Suzanne. *"We've had this argument before."* Suzanne nods, but Janet continues.

"You're darned right we have. She won't get a handicapped permit for her car."

Cindy looks up shyly. *"Well, most days I'm OK and I don't mind walking. Besides, I hate that staring. People are always checking you out to see if you really should be parking there."*

"That's hogwash. Why waste your energy? If you're having a good day, save yourself for when you're not feeling so well. Why should you walk three blocks and tire yourself out and

risk the consequences? Even when you're feeling good, why risk it?"

Cindy doesn't answer. But Janet is wound up and keeps at it.

"Like that business with your dog. Your physical therapist told you to go out and walk your dog in the morning. You said you'd do it, but I know you haven't."

"My dog is too big; I can't even hold him on a leash. He gets away from me. I even tripped over him once."

"Get a friend to go with you. She can hold the leash."

"Yeah, but I'm afraid I won't make it back and then she'll have me and the dog, and by that time people will be standing around gawking and I'll feel like a jerk."

Suzanne looks up after finishing the last of her fish.

"Look, I know what she means. People can be horrible. I'm caught in this kind of thing myself. My disability insurance has run out. Now that I've gotten better, they've decided that I'm no longer sick and I don't need disability. So I have to get a job. Do you know how hard that's going to be? I live in a small town; everyone knows who I am and that I have MS. They see me now and they think it's wonderful. But they've seen me when I couldn't stand up. You think someone's going to hire me? I'll answer that—they'll be too frightened that I'll have an attack and screw things up.

"I don't know what I'm going to do. But I know what Cindy means. People can be very, very cruel. If you don't have some support at home, and if you don't believe in yourself, then it can really get to you."

"Yep, you need a firm family base," Janet says as she swings around in her chair looking for the waiter. *"Not just your husband, but your kids. When I came back from Iowa I sat the kids down and told them: 'Sometimes Mommy's going to have to rest. Sometimes you'll have to be quiet. Sometimes Mommy will have to ask you to help her a little bit more.' They're not dumb, they got it. They actually kind of liked it— it gave them a little more responsibility around the house. It also made them feel good that I had thought they were old enough to explain it to them. I thought I should do it, though—not just for me, but for them. Otherwise I might be*

setting them up for ridicule by their friends. You know how kids ask, 'What's the matter with your mother?' That kind of thing."

Suzanne thinks for a moment and then shakes her head.

"You're right, Janet. My kids are older now. They can do more things for themselves, which we all like. When they were younger, though, I didn't handle it well. I wanted to do everything for them. It was a way of trying to avoid admitting that I was sick. There were days when I couldn't do all that I wanted to do, and I felt they suffered. I probably felt worse because I kept criticizing myself for what I couldn't do. That's silly. You shouldn't think like that. I was sure they thought less of me because I couldn't always be the perfect mom. It wasn't true, of course; they hardly noticed. You're doing the same thing, Cindy, giving other people much too much power over you."

Janet pipes up, busy with a fresh pot of tea.

"Right. Forget about those other people and start believing in yourself. Peter Samuels once told me a silly story about 'other people.' When he was in high school he had a teacher who was always telling him to do this or that. And Peter would always ask why. She would answer, 'Because they say so.' One day he asked her who 'they' were. She couldn't answer. He says he figured out if nobody knows who 'they' are, they can't be too important. Letting yourself be beaten down by a bunch of nameless faces, Cindy, you're crazy."

Psychologists and therapists consider that what we believe about ourselves and our capabilities can provide valuable clues to predicting our behavior. They suggest that people can build failure into their actions by their perceptions of the probable consequences of their efforts. This means that if a person believes that his actions may not produce positive or favorable results, there's a good chance they won't. Such beliefs may in turn initiate a chain of events to which failure is built in. Research has demonstrated, for example, that if an individual is able to adjust his behavior to cope with a difficult situation, the positive outcome will enhance his sense of self-worth.[1] Additionally, successful mastery over a difficult situation has been found to induce the confidence of being able to cope successfully with similar circumstances in the future. Who wouldn't want to face a difficult situation with the assurance that he's in control and can handle it?

On the other hand, if an individual doesn't cope appropriately, he is likely to experience a decrease in self-worth. This may produce a feeling opposite to one of control—a sinking feeling of helplessness. Not only does the person come to believe that he can't handle the situation; he can also end up feeling that it's gotten the best of him. The real danger is that he may generalize, or transmit, his belief of failure to other similar situations in the future, which will then cause additional failures and, finally, resignation to his perceived inability to cope.

People tend to function with two sets of beliefs in these matters. One relates to the individual's image of himself as a person; the other to his skills and capabilities. Often, a person who has difficulty managing risky situations, especially someone who is struggling with behavior such as overeating or alcoholism, tends to internalize his failures. Although it would seem to be best for him to step outside himself and analyze his behavior, he usually attributes his lack of success to a fundamental flaw in himself. He may completely ignore the fact that his behavior results from his interaction with his environment. The goal is to teach such people that their behavior is something they *do* rather than who they *are*.[2]

Obviously this school of thought is at odds with the common therapeutic approach of labeling people according to their addictive or consummatory behaviors. It would argue that calling someone a dope addict or an alcoholic provides a convenient crutch for the individual and may help program him to failure. The syndrome, they suggest, goes something like this: "I am an alcoholic; therefore, I possess the traits of an alcoholic. Unfortunately these traits make it difficult if not impossible for me to behave properly in certain situations which I define as high risk, specifically my ability to constrain myself in an occasion that might offer me the opportunity of taking a drink. If I take that drink, it could lead me to take too many drinks, so I should stay out of those situations."

The trouble with the latter approach is that although—as

we've seen—it is possible to change behavior, it is all but impossible to change a trait, and that's what the above individual is blaming his problems on—a personality trait. What is a trait anyhow? What does it look like? How would you go about changing it? What will it look like when you're finished?

A trait is fundamentally a descriptive abstraction, which we often think of as responsible for behavior; i.e., we might say of a person, "It is a trait of his to be antagonistic to strangers." You notice that in describing the trait we are describing the person's behavior. So it is the behavior that should be observed and evaluated and on which an individual should focus his efforts. He will need to change his actions so that they are responsive to his need for coping with his problematic situations. In doing so, he would have something tangible to work toward as well as benchmarks on which to evaluate attainment of his goals.

We can apply some of this logic to the problems of multiple sclerosis. The difference between Janet's and Cindy's attitudes is based in their perception of themselves. Cindy has taken MS as part of her identity in the way an alcoholic accepts his label. Janet has not. Although Janet necessarily has to consider her affliction when planning and executing certain aspects of her life, her concern is with her *actions* rather than her self-concept. This has enabled her to remain active, living her life with the same spirit and verve as before she discovered the MS. She handles the disease as a factor that may present her with a variety of new and difficult situations, but one to which she can apply her abilities and come out smelling like a rose. She has learned the necessity of developing and implementing new coping strategies. Perhaps, most importantly, she has not subjugated her identity to the fact of her illness. She is still fundamentally Janet, facing the challenges that life deals her.

On the other hand, Cindy seems to have accepted the MS label and has become preoccupied with how people will react to her new identity. She wastes valuable time reacting to what she sees as their response, rather than developing behavior to cope with the situations that will logically result from her MS. On one hand, she has tried to deny her disease with overwork and defiance. On the other hand, she succumbs to it by directly confronting situations for which she is unprepared and which strengthen her feelings of inadequacy.

Other factors that can influence our behavior involve the messages we formulate about ourselves and our actions. We often translate these messages into commands, along with our thoughts and daydreams about ourselves. Psychologists refer to these self-directed messages as *self-speech*. These can further be divided into three parts: self-instructions, classifications, and beliefs.[3] Self-instructions are obvious. They are the commands or orders we all routinely give ourselves. Some we are aware of at various levels of consciousness, others we're not. These may include such diverse messages as "I need to go to the grocery store before the beginning of the week" and "Look out for this corner; there's usually a lot of traffic." Because they often appear at a subconscious level, we are not always aware of the content of these self-instructions.

Without realizing it, a person with MS can be doing himself in with his self-instructions. If you're confused or uncomfortable about your MS, your self-instructions may be geared to avoiding situations in which you feel you can't perform—such as Cindy's walking her dog. If such were the case, your job would be to sit down and listen to yourself, making notes about the commands you issue, so you can see where they're taking you. If you're on top of things, as Janet is, monitoring your commands to yourself would probably leave you pleased with how well you're doing. Obviously, if you're unhappy with the way things are shaping up, if you feel tentative and shy because of your MS, you will want to change your self-instructions.

Our classification of ourselves—as competent or special or inadequate—can also affect our behavior and its subsequent outcome. Likewise our evaluation of the character of the situations in which we find ourselves, as challenging or neutral or a piece of cake, as well as our view of how other people perceive us. So, because of a few bad experiences,

Cindy might classify grocery shopping as a situation that causes her difficulty, amplifying her problem with the subconscious description "Oh, no, here it comes again. I have to buy groceries. The last time I did that there was that awful woman. I'll send Ron instead." Or, even worse, "I'll never sit in that wheelchair again because I don't want another person asking me why I can't walk."

Suzanne's self-classification that she's unemployable because of her MS is going to make looking for a job an enterprise fraught with frustration and failure. She should direct her energy toward developing a positive strategy for her job search. Otherwise she is just priming herself to fulfill her self-prediction—she won't find a job. Additionally, if she classifies herself as a poor risk, think of what she will be projecting to potential employers. She should think of the job search as an exciting and interesting process, an opportunity for self-fulfillment, as well as a job. To do this she will probably need to change her perception of her job skills.

The final category of self-speech is perhaps the most significant because it entails our own belief system, which may be so well hidden that we are barely aware of it. We probably use it for a basis of action almost every day. Suzanne, for example, is inhibiting herself with her belief that employers in her community won't hire her because she has MS. Incidentally, this conviction is not based on any direct experience, but rather on what she thinks people's reaction will be. Equally destructive is Cindy's belief that people will think badly of her if she is not able to perform as well as she thinks they think she should.

What both women fail to realize is that it is they who are imposing the standards and attributing them to other people. Cindy also has fallen into the trap of unjustifiably transferring a generalization from one situation to many others. As we have indicated, inappropriate behavior in one situation doesn't mean you are doomed forever. This happens only if you take one instance of your behavior and sanctify it as a belief about yourself. It is doubtful that Cindy has asked her neighbors what they think about her walking her dog. If she were to do so, it's likely that she might find a different reaction than she anticipates and would probably find a friend to help her.

To correct this situation, an individual would have to implement a strategy similar to those for his changing self-instructions and his classification system. He would have to listen to himself, identify his self-beliefs, perhaps even write them down and then scrutinize them for validity. Interestingly enough, the psychologists tell us that, as individuals in this society, our two most common beliefs (to which MS victims seem to be particularly vulnerable) are: (1) that the constant love and approval of those around us is desirable and necessary; and (2) that everything we do must be executed to perfection.[4] Before we go any further, let us state uncategorically that both of these beliefs are invalid.

Sadly, a person with MS could come to believe that he is less lovable because of his disease. He might also succumb to a diminishing sense of self-worth because he can no longer perform on a level he considers acceptable. Forget both. Nobody is lovable all the time, every day, under every circumstance; nor is it physically possible always to act in a way that will generate approval from the great variety of people with whom most of us routinely interact. Most people's standards of perfection are idealized, based in part on their erroneous perception of their past performance. It would be unreasonable for Cindy or Janet or Suzanne or anyone else to compare their capabilities as an MS patient with themselves before MS. They are dealing with a totally different set of circumstances. If you will remember our discussion in Chapter 9 about adhering to an allergy-free diet, it is the harmonious adaptation of your actions to the circumstances in which you find yourself that generates happiness.

Three recommendations are made. First, listen to what you tell yourself about yourself and about the circumstances in which you might routinely interact. Also be aware of your beliefs about your ability to cope with your various potentially troublesome situations. It would then make sense to jot down some of your observations and allow yourself a couple of quiet hours to reflect on what you've uncovered. What basis do you have, for example, for your belief that as a person with MS you are limited in one way or another? From where do you derive that belief—by talking to other people? Who? How are they managing their lives—are they lives of expanding opportunity or of closing options? Did you read it somewhere? If so, the same questions apply: Who wrote it? What is his perspective on life? How is he managing? Did a health professional suggest it? Have you tested these conclusions in real life, in your own life? Have you matched your experience with theirs? Were there incongruities? Do you have faith in your experience or are you relying on that of others? You could be just as much of an expert, especially when it comes to yourself and your expectations. Do you consider yourself incapacitated by MS in some way? Exactly how? What situations have you identified as giving you problems—appearing in public, inconveniencing others, meeting new people, accomplishing something independently?

Now look at what you say to yourself about these situations. Are you conditioning yourself with a negative message such as "I know I inconvenience my friends by going to their house for dinner because my wheelchair won't fit under the dining room table and they have to move things around for me, so I won't go," or "I know my mother doesn't like to go shopping with me anymore because some days I move slowly, so I'm not going to ask her again. It will save her from being embarrassed."?

Have you ever asked your friend or her husband about whether it bothers her to clear an extra space at the table? Have you spoken to your mother about whether or not she truly thinks you're slow and, better yet, whether she cares? Perhaps she would rather have your company than not. You should consider verifying these beliefs by directly asking the people about your fears and concerns. Only then will you be able to dispel the demons you're creating for yourself. There may be an occasional person out there who really doesn't have the capability to rise to the occasion of another person's illness. But they are few and far between, and you should not generalize based on an occasional unfortunate experience.

If you talk to the people whom you credit with your

erroneous beliefs and expose your misconceptions, you can then use that information to change your instructions to yourself. In the case of your friend, instead of saying, "They don't want me and my wheelchair at dinner," you would say, "I'm going to go to the party and talk to everyone and have a wonderful time. They wouldn't ask me if they didn't want me." Or, about your mother, think, "I really enjoy the time we spend together, and I think she does also. It's one way she can feel like she's helping me."

It may take a while to sort out these self-generated thoughts, but don't despair. Take Cindy, for example. Although she is still struggling with her preoccupation with other people's concerns about her, she mastered one essential area for herself and has done something about it. She evaluated her own view of what was going to happen to her as a result of her MS diagnosis and decided that she didn't believe she would end up in a wheelchair like her grandfather. And you know what? She hasn't. But she may be compromising her chances of staying up and around if she doesn't alter some of her other beliefs about her illness, especially about the effects of her appearance and actions on others, particularly strangers, who probably give her less thought than she gives them.

"Talk to yourself" is what the experts advise, particularly if you occasionally find yourself in a sticky situation.[5] Your self-instructions should concern not just your actions but also your beliefs about yourself and the circumstances of your MS. If you find that in a crowded room your behavior is motivated by the belief that people are offended or inconvenienced by your presence, manufacture a different set of instructions, such as "Hey, listen, I know this is a scary situation, but really you're a pretty bright person, and I bet most of those people would like to talk to you. Now go to it." It's OK to get outside of yourself and engage in conversation with you. It helps you adopt a detached perspective about yourself, your beliefs, and the labels you may have erroneously accepted.

This brings us back to where we started—other people. We've already discussed your beliefs about them, but what about their beliefs about you? Do you even know what they believe? Your job is to discover what they think and correct it if it's wrong. Suzanne says that MS people and the people around them need education. By this she means information about what multiple sclerosis is about and what to expect. But you also have to know what your family and close friends believe about your illness and about you now that you have it. This is particularly important if you think their perception of you has changed. Suzanne's husband thought about divorce. Perhaps he believed that she was going to become incapacitated and said to himself, "You'd better get out while you can. This may be a situation you won't be able to handle." Such thoughts necessarily relate to his own beliefs about himself. Under such circumstances his instructions could have been, "I can't handle this, especially if she gets worse, which I guess maybe she might, so maybe I'd better evaluate my options."

On the other hand, someone like Janet's husband, Nat, would seem to have a different outlook. He not only believed that MS could be licked but that Janet had the courage and skill to do it. His charge to himself would seem to have been: "This is a situation in which you can win; go out and do it. Help her."

It is extremely important that your spouse understand the nature of your disease, its probable consequences, and how you're planning to deal with it. Research shows that lack of reinforcement from others can have a very specific, negative effect on a person's efforts to cope. It has been found, for example, that people in psychological therapy who are not supported for the changes they make as a result of that therapy often don't complete it.[6] You don't want that to happen to you—you don't want others to discourage you from your own attempts to help yourself.

If you're engaged in efforts at self managed change—to stick to your diet and stay healthy—you will require all the help you can get. The last thing you need is for someone to be negative, especially someone as important to you as your spouse. Therapists tell us that in a strained relationship, as might happen when an individual is diagnosed with MS, a crucial strategy is to listen to each other and be polite (married couples are known to be ruder to each other than to co-workers in similar situations).[7] In addition, you both need to be willing to compromise, to express your feelings, and to expect the same of the other person. Open communication, in a few words, is the ticket.

Start the process yourself, and if you find you're not getting as far as you'd like, then seek professional help. If you're uncomfortable seeing a therapist, perhaps your physician could aid you; maybe a close friend who could listen to both sides and mediate a compromise. The important thing is to do something. It's not productive for you to be hanging out there without any support, and you can't possibly relish the idea of your spouse's being confused and frustrated by what's happening to you. Peter Samuels has spoken considerably about the difficulties a spouse may feel when he or she discovers the partner has MS. He likened it to an appliance that arrives new but broken. He's right—the immediate reaction is often to send it back. Probably a reason to feel that way is because there appears to be no way to fix it. The only solution, if you are ill with a condition that can affect not only yourself but your whole household, is to inform them of what's going on. Likewise you need to apprise them about what you're expecting of yourself and of them. You don't need the kids to scream, "Oh, no, not chicken again," when you're doing your best to forget that you haven't had a steak in months. After all, they can sneak out and have a burger. You're stuck with the poultry.

It's important that your family and friends understand and cope with the situation so that they can act in both your and their best interests. And everybody in your family should stop and think a minute—if they're having trouble coping with your MS, they should think about what it's doing to you.

One excellent way to deal with the challenge of the other people in your life is to get them involved in your projects.[8] During the time you're attempting to identify those potentially dangerous situations that might cause you to eat the foods to which you're allergic, ask your spouse and perhaps your children to help you identify possible pitfalls. Aside from the fact that it will introduce them to the process, they could have insights into your behavior that you don't. Once you determine what those situations are, involve your family in your efforts to adhere to your program. You might ask them to remind you of your goals, especially in circumstances you've identified as potentially difficult for you.

It could be as simple as telling you to watch what you eat when you go to a certain restaurant because they have the best cheesecake in town and you love cheesecake but you're on a nondairy diet. Language, especially the language of others, is considered to have one of the strongest and most immediate effects on our behavior. Obviously, you wouldn't want your family reminders to become heavy-handed or intimidating. What you are looking for is a gentle reminder. The group should also be available to praise you when you make it through a tight situation and for you to brag to about your accomplishments. Any such arrangements should be made beforehand so you all know the rules. Yours are to stick to the goals of your new program; theirs are to help you do it.

Just as MS patients can be confused and frustrated by the thought of not being able to do anything about their disease, spouses are not strangers to such feelings. Give your spouse an opportunity to help. He or she will feel better for it. Your spouse might even become your assistant—the one who holds the reward money or helps you evaluate whether or not you've completed what you were striving for. He or she might keep the records and require you to report. Again, in any of these cases your spouse could be a real help to you and, in the process, learn about what you're doing and what it means. Clearly, the most effective key to understanding among people is, and always has been, information. You may have to take the lead, but do it. On the other hand, spouses can provide auxiliary reinforcement of their own making. A present, a special kiss, an unexpected weekend away can help show you that your spouse thinks you're right on the money and can be wonderfully motivating. Such surprises can be a pleasant replacement if you've had to give up something—like your favorite food. You even might want him or her to share your reward. Do something with your spouse that you might not ordinarily make time for. That way, if you miss your mark, you've disappointed not only yourself but also your partner.

What you accomplish with your husband or wife or the most important individual in your life you should, of course, carry through with everyone who is close to you. You may occasionally have the need to use a friend or relative for a little shoulder crying, as Suzanne did. Her friendships with other MS patients helped her get through that difficult period when her husband was confused and thought he wanted a divorce. There is one thing you should always remember: most people want to help, but they don't always know the best way. Give your friends and family a break and tell them what you need.

There's no doubt that people stare and that you could use others as your point of reference about MS if you wanted. But that would be foolhardy. They don't have your disease. Furthermore, it's not their life; it's yours. You have to cope with your MS. You have to determine what you believe about yourself as a person afflicted with multiple sclerosis. Other people should never inhibit you from being the best you can be; but you should consider them as potential helpers in the process.

Take heed of Janet's words: *"I told myself I was going to beat this thing. I wasn't stupid enough to let it go at that and trust to blind chance. I took the precaution of telling myself that I had the skills to win the battle, and what I didn't have I was going to go and get."*

You can't beat that for strategy.

12

PHYSICAL THERAPY—
ANOTHER ESSENTIAL

Cindy Morse is staring across the room at Janet Myerson, who is doing an exercise that makes her look like she's practicing to throw out the first ball of the World Series. Janet peers back at her. *"What's the matter, Cindy? You look upset."*

"I was just thinking; some people have all the luck."

Janet stops what she's doing. *"What do you mean?"*

Cindy is a little embarrassed by her outburst, but she continues. *"Like you. Your doctor was a family friend; your physical therapist comes to your house. Some people just get all the breaks."*

"Come on, Cindy. My first doctor—our so-called family friend—did absolutely nothing for my MS, except put me in the hospital to be tested and questioned for hundreds of dollars a day. My therapist comes to the house because I called and asked him. I convinced him that I needed him and that I couldn't do it without him, plus I promised that I'd do what he told me. You have to do these things for yourself. There's no silver platter. Life isn't like that, whether you have MS or you don't."

180

Common wisdom aside, people are not generally born with the knowledge to survive or contrarily, with a predilection for destruction. We learn such things, and having learned one or the other, we can unlearn it. Learning, of course, does not refer exclusively to the act of sitting down with the express purpose of acquiring some kind of knowledge or skill. We "learn" things based on our environment and its pressures and the people with whom we live and their life-styles and perspectives. The experts, however, do tell us that the key to a productive life is simple: balance. Ah, you say, a lovely thought, but what does it mean?[1]

Balance in living means keeping our efforts consistent and evenly distributed. One recommendation is to divide our activities into three areas. One-third of our time and effort should be earmarked for a job or some form of professional development. One-third is for our family and friends, and one-third is for pleasurable activities that we should find fulfilling. Obviously a job or some kind of work is necessary for survival. Additionally, most people have responsibilities involving family and friends. We all know, however, that work is never all work—most of us obtain some enjoyment from it, as well as from our interaction with friends and relatives. However, the final third of our effort—fulfill-ment—is meant to be a release from those things we per-ceive as "what we are supposed to do." The point is that a little change of perspective and effort is good for what may ail you. Even better, consider it an investment in preventive maintenance, instead of waiting until you're stuck in a breakdown to straighten things out.

What we all should strive for is a proper ratio between the *should-dos* and *would-like-tos* of life. The should-dos are those activities we perceive as generated by outside de-mands or pressures. It is not that we might not choose to do them in the first place, but that our perception of the activity makes it something we should do, often for the benefit of others. It is, if you will, a responsibility. The would-like-tos are those things we perceive as pleasurable and fulfilling and are undertaken under our own volition and often for our own exclusive benefit.

If your life gets tipped too far toward the shoulds, it is predictable that you will come to feel "overloaded," perhaps even oppressed. The next step is to sink into feeling sorry for yourself. At this point you may be susceptible to doing something crazy. Hopefully, it won't be of the caliber of jumping from a bridge, but it could involve sneaking off for some kind of little indulgence which you feel will reduce your feeling of oppression. This is the stage at which the alcoholic may take a drink, the drug-addicted individual reach for the medicine chest, or the overweight person splurge on hot fudge sundaes. Indeed, it has been argued that people who struggle with consummatory behavior often discover their lives to be horribly overburdened with should-dos and terribly bankrupt of would-like-tos.

If you provision your life with shoulds, they will eventually get you. Perhaps without knowing it, you will attempt to cope by instituting your chocolate cake in the afternoon or two martinis before dinner. The difficulty is that such strategies are not ultimately fulfilling; in fact, they usually generate subsequent negative feelings. First of all, people often end up feeling guilty about their splurges, often chastising themselves for their weakness. Second, they are forced to expend additional time and energy on the repair process—getting back on the wagon or losing the three extra pounds they gained in chocolate. The result can be the addition of more shoulds to an already overloaded system.

The hopeful aspect of this syndrome is, as we suggested earlier, that you can change your should-dos to would-like-tos by changing your perspective. A young woman we know liked exercise, truly enjoyed it. Being a perfectionist, she set up an elaborate program to ensure that she kept to her schedule. She went faithfully to the gym six times a week, whether she felt like it or not. Two things happened. First, she started hating her exercise. It went from something she wanted to do to something she had to do. She experienced considerable anxiety when it appeared that she might not be able to get to the gym, and she suffered if her performance fell below what she had established as her standard.

The second result was that because she became so compulsive about her routine, she ended up overtraining. Chained to her rule that she had to exercise even when she didn't feel like it, she frequently ended up ill and unable to train. In desperation, she finally consulted an exercise physiologist who explained to her that she was overtraining. He also insisted that she take time off if she didn't feel up to par. She joined another club that designed a program for her, starting slowly (far below the level she thought she should be at) and working up so that she could manage her routine without anxiety. The attitude of her new, more well-informed instructors was informal and relaxed, which enabled her to remove the should from her exercise and get back to enjoying it.

It must be obvious to you that, as a person with MS, you could become particularly susceptible to the shoulds. If you give yourself a chance, you could probably build up a should list long enough to trip over. This is partly the result of the fact that as an MS victim you may have a more than usual need to perform your should-do behavior. This is probably because you want to demonstrate your capabilities, which is in turn related to your concern that some day, or week, or month you might not be able to do so. Being able to carry out your perceived responsibilities also provides you with a benchmark to use as proof that you're not in such bad shape after all. Such concerns are also probably involved with the opinions of others—you may be reasoning that, if people see that you're still able to discharge your duties, then perhaps they won't write you off because of MS.

So, typically, many MS patients add a disproportionate amount of should-dos to their lives. They may feel they have to push themselves harder, to prove themselves because of their disease. Or they may reach further on the days they feel good against the days they may not feel so fit. The problem is that this compulsion for success could detract from the activities they establish to control their MS. If a person attacks his new lifestyle program armed with a collection of shoulds, he's setting himself up for failure. Strapped into his determination not to let MS get him, he may end up translating what could be wants into shoulds, tipping his life into negative balance.

Thus far, we have attempted to explain that being too strict with yourself can be counterproductive. We have talked about willpower and how it is better to develop coping strategies rather than hard and fast rules. We have shown how you can eat reasonably and still control your MS. We have asked you not to suffer alone, but to seek the help, support, guidance, and counsel of others. Now we have one more thing we'd like you to do: exercise. Oh, yes, one other thing—try to think of it as a would-like-to rather than a should-do. We want you to do this because exercise, aside from its obvious physiological benefits, also provides an outlet for frustration and tension. This in turn can be a great asset to you in establishing a balanced lifestyle.

Physiologically speaking, everyone needs exercise. We Americans all seem to eat too much and do too little. We run into health problems associated with this out-of-balance equation—from heart disease, which is still at the top of our list of killers, down through diabetes, hypertension, gout, and plain old obesity, which, if left to itself long enough, can lead to other problems. Every muscle of your body, including your heart, needs to be stressed in order to work properly. An MS patient needs exercise for all the usual reasons and more.

As with many of the other problems associated with MS, your exercise problems can start at diagnosis. First of all, you've probably been laid up in the hospital for a week or so. You may not have been very active up to that point because of the MS. Then you go home, generally feeling pretty defeated and under the weather. As Janet Myerson suggested, you would not be blamed for the urge to shut yourself inside the walls of your bedroom to scream. Emotionally this may seem like the least likely time to start an exercise program. Actually it's the best time to get going, before your physical as well as emotional load gets too heavy. Janet succumbed to the weight of her illness and stayed in bed until she came back from Waterloo. The spark was ignited in the Waterloo hospital, where they forced her to go down to the physical therapy unit even though she didn't feel up to it. Janet remembers her Waterloo experience:

"I came right home from Waterloo and called Ian and barked, 'Come right over here. I need help.' He did, and sometimes I ask myself, 'Why did I do that?' All that stretching and pulling and sweating. But you have to do it. You see, what MS patients don't realize is that you forget how to do things.

"If you've been in the hospital for a while, your joints are stiff and all that, but let's face it, what do you do in the hospital? Nothing. You lie there. You don't fix dinner, you don't do the laundry, you don't type or file or answer or dial a telephone or sew on a button. My God, you don't even get dressed. You're just there.

"One thing I was shocked about was how much I'd forgotten. I figured that Ian and I would start out with the big stuff, walking between parallel bars, calisthenics in the living room, that kind of thing. How wrong could I have been? What we started with was learning how to button my clothes, how to hold a fork—better yet, how to get the fork to my mouth. Changing diapers, holding on to a spatula so I could cook. For some mysterious reason, your fingers forget how to bend. Have you ever thought of the things you do that require you to bend your fingers? I mean I couldn't even pick up a toothbrush. Ugh.

"I'm grateful for Ian. I don't know whether I would have gotten as strong as I did if he hadn't come faithfully every Saturday. I always complained, and he'd just smile and say, 'Work harder, Come on, work harder.' "

There are a number of special characteristics to Janet's physical therapy program. During her stay in the Waterloo hospital she experienced the benefit of personal cooperation between herself and the therapist. This, she says, helped encourage her to pursue a program of therapy when she got home. Back in Philadelphia, however, Ian added two other factors: he worked with her to develop the kind of patterned movement she would need to get herself completely in shape, and he designed a program that integrated her therapy into her lifestyle.

Let's start with the latter first. It could be that physical therapy has acquired a bad rap. The words themselves evoke the image of a cold, depersonalizing process, basically a stupifying and perhaps boring activity effectively similar to taking one's medicine. Another view suggests tedious days spent in constantly repeating artificial movements seemingly designed by someone with no knowledge of the needs and desires of human beings. Endless hours sweating away in a dank, padded room, only to emerge with "skills" that seem to have very little to do with the rest of your life.

Janet's therapist chose the living room for their sessions. The front room is the center of activity in the Myerson household, and because of this, Janet originally suggested they use the den or a bedroom for their work. Ian insisted on the living room, however, only to end up playing horse with Janet's children and dodging the family pets.

"We used to have a joke of the week," Janet explains. *"Ian would come dashing into the house, and the kids would run up to him, yelling 'Tell us, tell us.' Sometimes they were funny, but most of the time they weren't. Obviously, it was the ritual that counted."*

Ian's jokes and his living room therapy had the effect of involving the whole family in the process of Janet's rehabilitation. They knew what she was doing, and they understood why she was doing it. And she knew that they knew; this helped her keep to her program. Initially at least, this family interaction facilitated the "assistance" problem. The virtues and consequences of assigning an MS patient a cane or walker or even a wheelchair have been debated over and over, among patients, physicians, and therapists. One view holds that there are times when a person is so weak that he should use whatever help he can get. The argument continues that it is better to use some form of assistance and get out in the world than to risk staying home and easing further into the debilitating effects of MS. The opposite view suggests that using assistance is equivalent to giving in to the disease and starts the inevitable downhill spiral that will end in a wheelchair or bed.

Ian managed a practical compromise between the two views. The basis of his therapy in this regard is that there will be times when any individual may not be up to par—perhaps as a result of an exacerbation, perhaps because of overdoing. In such cases, however, it is best that the individual not decide to sit down and wait it out. This only makes the return to activity that much more difficult. Muscles get weak; coordination deteriorates. In such situations a person should take advantage of assistance to get around, so he doesn't risk losing whatever gains he's accumulated. The secret, however, is to do so in a manner that won't interfere with subsequent progress, either physically or emotionally.

If a patient feels the need of assistance, Ian suggests using something of a temporary nature. This eliminates the negativity frequently associated with buying a cane or walker or especially a wheelchair. Use walls, for example. Walk around your living room and practice using the walls for balance. Run your hand against the wall. Don't lean; just use it for balance and support. This is a good strategy when your legs feel weak. When you reach the point that you feel comfortable about walking around the periphery of the room, then take a chance and cut across it, walking back and forth between the walls. Then when you go out and feel the need for support, all you have to do is reach for the nearest wall. It really is a very natural gesture, similar to hanging on to a railing or a banister, which is why they were put there in the first place.

A second helping device is another person's arm. Ian explains:

"I knew a person once who was partially blind because of diabetes. He had lost the sight in one eye and was subject to periods when the sight in his other eye failed because of rupturing blood vessels. This man was a young, high-powered businessman. It would hardly do for him to walk around with a cane. This certainly wasn't in his self-image. He was very cool about how he handled the situation. He'd walk into a room and pinpoint where everyone was by their voices. Then he'd head right on in and shake hands. He could see shapes, so he didn't run into tables or chairs, and he would just proceed to feel his way along a wall or the conference table. If he had to move quickly or was in unknown territory,

he might take the arm of the person nearest him, asking permission with his head bent to the person's ear. If you were a woman, it would be a full-fledged gesture—he'd slide his arm through yours. Most women were highly flattered. He might put his arm on a man's shoulder and ask quietly if he could walk next to him until they reached the top of the stairs. Nobody thought a thing of it, and he was able to get through periods when he was almost completely blind without people realizing there was something drastically wrong. Imagine how an individual such as he would have suffered if he'd had to walk with a cane or some other kind of device.

"So I tell people to take someone's arm, maybe your husband's or a friend's. I think this is infinitely better than the strategy another friend of mine used. He had a rare back ailment that caused him a great deal of pain. He had to walk with a cane because he couldn't stand up straight and was often weak from all the medication he took. He was another one of those dynamic businessmen, however, who prided himself on out-strategizing the opposition and dealing from a position of strength. In his mind, it would never have worked for him to come stumbling into a meeting with a cane. So he didn't. He'd hobble up to the door with his various lieutenants following behind, carrying his files and briefcase. Then he'd hand the cane to an assistant, throw open the door, and stride into the room like a conquering general. I bet those few moments of 'glory' cost him an inordinate amount of physical and mental effort."

The message, then, is to use assistance if you have to, but do not feel strapped to something that may cause you negative repercussions. Use the things that are already in your life. Few people will even notice. The corollary to that, however, is *don't overdo*, so that your only option is a wheelchair. Also, practice your assistance strategies, so you'll have them handy when you need them. Do things gradually. If you've just gotten home from the hospital, and you want to work back into things again, do it slowly. Set your marks at intervals; practice until you can routinely meet your mark and then move up.

Cindy, for example, might start her walks without her dog.

Forget the dog, and think of first things first. What, for example, would she have to do if she were to take the dog for a spin around the block? Initially, she'd have to get out of the house, then down the front steps, then down her sidewalk to the street. So what she should do first is practice getting out the door and walking down the steps to the end of her property and back. She should do this for a week or two or for whatever time is required until she feels strong.

The objective is to establish a routine so there are no questions and no excuses about your activity. If you feel the need for measurement, then say to yourself, "I want to walk five hundred feet unaided. It's about five hundred feet to my mailbox. OK, that's my goal. Every day for the next two weeks, right after lunch, I'll go out and get the mail."

The idea is that you slowly build up your muscles and get the juices going again. Incidentally, you're not alone in this. Anyone who starts an exercise program must start gradually. Even the best athletes don't start off running 26 miles if they've never run before. Everyone does need exercise, however. As Ian says:

"Even if you suffer from MS, you're just not using up all your energy waking up in the morning and walking to the bathroom. I don't care how bad or weak you feel. You've got more than that in you. It may take time to get going, but the human body is made for work. Your MS may interfere with your coordination because of short circuits in your nervous system. But your muscles still have the capacity to work. For that, you need practice to build up your muscle strength and to regain coordination. Keeping the muscle structure strong so that you can accomplish routine tasks with a minimum of effort provides your body with extra stamina to fight the allergic reaction that underlies MS.

"There's just so much you can do; however, if your muscles are weak, it's going to take twice as much energy to get around. If you've got any kind of motivation at all, and you do too much, you'll end up wearing yourself down. You risk getting an infection and then your immunological system, which may be weak in the first place, doesn't get the support it needs, and you're back in that vicious cycle."

So Ian came every Saturday to Janet's house, whether she liked it or not, and gave her the benchmarks to achieve. Aside from his expertise as a physical therapist, Janet says he helped her immensely as someone to talk to.

"He knew about the disease. I could ask him all those questions I couldn't ask anyone else. I didn't feel so alone. He would answer the stupid questions I'd be afraid to ask, say, of my doctor. I felt like here was someone really interested in what was happening to me as a person. The therapists at the hospital in Waterloo were like that, although I wasn't really in much shape to take advantage of them then. I was still so weak. They had just put me on the diet, and my mind wasn't working that well. But they dragged me down there every day, just like everyone else. The therapists seemed to know a lot about MS. They pushed us, and I know they talked to Dr. Soll about us if we didn't go as far as we were supposed to. They would recommend things to him about how much further we could and should go.

"That's why I think that physical therapy is important. You can't see your doctor once a week, and even if you could, your time would be limited. Besides, the interaction is formal; it's hard to really discuss something. When you're rolling around the floor or practicing how to lift your legs you can talk informally. Having Ian come each week was a reminder that I still had to work on this thing and that I still could. It was another aspect of hope."

Ian agrees.

"I tell my patients, 'I'm not leaving; I'm here for the duration, until you get through the exercises the way I know you can do them.' You listen to a lot of problems, like how their family is or isn't accepting their MS. You try to second-guess them a little bit—to see if they're really accepting it like they say they are. You need to be able to determine whether it's a great show and they're just churning inside, because if that's the case, then you can predict they won't do well with their therapy.

"I guess the most difficult thing to listen to—because you can't do much about it—is the constant fear that tomorrow they're going to get worse. I've had some people give it to me

straight out: 'Look, I've got this disease. I believe I can get worse any minute, so I'm going to give up, because it just isn't worth it.' That's when you really have to push. The other thing a physical therapist can do that a physician or family members can't is listen to a patient's war stories. You ask them what happened, why they think it happened, and what they think they can do to prevent it from happening again."

Ian's treatment for Janet was a whole-body approach.

"When a person gets to the point where he or she is feeling fairly good, then it's time to strengthen his or her entire musculature. I don't believe in exercising just the legs or the arms or whatever seems to be the immediate problem, because then you've got a strong part dragging a weak part, and you're back with wasting a lot of energy. The whole body has to be strong. If the person's arms are OK or doing well, then we'll push him a little further. If the legs are what seem to be the problem, I'll take my time and make sure the patient has something for that, too, but we'd also be working the arms at the same time. If you ignore the rest of the body in favor of the explicit problem the patient is having at the time, then you're just buying trouble later on down the line.

"First, we work on the upper extremities and then the lower extremities, and then we work on trunk motions: side-side, forward and back, crawling, resisted walking. I use a lot of patterned exercises because I'm convinced that they provide input into the nervous system. What we work with is patterns that simulate normal movement. There are groups of muscles that are required to work together in a specific format, so to speak. You may use similar patterns to throw a ball, pick up a magazine, take something down from a cupboard, or hug your child. It's like practicing any sport. You practice so that when the time comes you don't have to think about the basic motions that are involved in what you have to do.

"I've seen what can happen if you put someone on a program of strict, seemingly meaningless exercises. They resent them. They don't see any use for them, and they don't do them. Sometimes they even get angry at me. I can see they're thinking to themselves, 'Who is this turkey who's

telling me I have to do these stupid exercises three times a day, ten times each?' I proceed on the basis that everybody enjoys some kind of physical activity—running, walking, swimming, riding a bike, whatever. I try to get them in shape for it, and then I help them put together a program for their favorite sport."

Physical therapy, as Janet experienced it, is unfortunately not always available to patients. According to the usual pattern, the physician will assign the patient to therapy while he or she is in the hospital. The prescription is usually very specific and will be followed right down to the last detail by the therapist. Doctor and therapist usually have little interaction. Physical therapy is not a field the physician knows intimately; he is busy enough with his own area of expertise. It appears that the main thrust of physical therapy, unless you are in an innovative program or have a therapist like Ian, is to target minimum, as opposed to maximum, gains. This is at least partially related to the fact that the cost of physical therapy is usually covered by health insurance. Schedules are established which reflect the goal of specific and immediate progress, as opposed to the type of maintenance program that might help the patient preserve what movement he currently has and prevent him from sliding. The result is that a standard health insurance policy would not pay for a program like Janet's. Physicians know this, so when they send their prescription to the physical therapy department, they are likely to go for a specific, although minimum, goal. A doctor's request is likely to be something like, "Please get this patient to the point at which she can ambulate with a walker." If the therapist were to come back to the physician and tell him that he thinks he can push the patient further, he is not likely to be greeted with enthusiasm.

This problem is complicated by the fact that, in most states, a therapist needs a prescription from a physician to treat a patient. So, aside from the fact that the therapist can't operate independently, he is also not free to prescribe a program beyond what the physician has authorized. Occasionally a therapist can lobby for another month or two of therapy, but that is usually all. Everyone is aware of how the system works, and no one wants to be caught abusing it. It is a sad but fundamentally true fact that once a patient levels off in gains, there will be no more money from the insurance company to pay for physical therapy, regardless of the fact that this might be the point at which the patient needs it most.

If an individual does not pay close attention during therapy, or the therapist hasn't taken the time to work with the patient's family, the entire exercise may end up a waste of time. The patient will fall off his program and into the inevitable slide.

So we are again up against another case in which the MS patient has to take the initiative. This may require working with his physician to develop a program of maximum gains for the exercise portion of his treatment program. It may require the time and energy of both the patient and the physician to locate a therapist who will help meet the goals of maintenance therapy. It may take some creative accounting on everyone's part, or it may require a dip into the patient's own pocketbook.

But whatever it takes, it is worth it. It will compromise your efforts in modifying other areas of your lifestyle if you sit around in a cloud of physical sloth. Watching your diet, and trying to stay out of the way of infection and fatigue will not be as effective if you neglect to implement an exercise program. So why risk it? You've put in a lot of effort thus far. We're only asking you to do little bit more. Remember the secret.

Balance.

13

SUMMARIZING
THE SOLL TREATMENT

"I know what it's like for me and for the other patients I've talked to. The thing that gets me to do what I should do is that I've gotten better."

Peter Samuels is sitting in the conference room of the MS clinic in Waterloo, warming his hands around a mug of tea. Suzanne Baccone watches him across the table as she twirls the ends of her hair between two fingers.

"Listen,"she says, "Dr. Soll said to me, 'Let's just start out by trying to keep you at your present level. We may not be able to make you better, but let's at least keep you from getting worse.' I told him that was OK with me. At that point I wasn't thinking about the future in terms of getting back any of what I had lost; I just didn't want to get worse. It's taken a little work, but I've not only maintained that level, I'm a lot better than I was when I started."

"You were lucky, Suzanne; you happened to be in the right place at the right time,"responds Peter. "You got the systematic treatment. As someone who came later, you benefited from the work Dr. Soll did with people like me. When I first started we didn't know about food allergies. The big thing

194

was trying to control the symptoms, in the hope of decreasing the possibility that they would get worse. There was also some thought given to the role of infection. Those were the early days, when we were attempting to sort things out. I am certainly happy that I was a part of that time. If you went to see Dr. Soll then—he was at the university at the time—you'd get antibiotics for the infection. I have to admit that sometimes I didn't even know I had an infection; sloppy, I was very sloppy back then. Of course I also didn't know about endotoxin, so if I had had an infection, I probably wouldn't have paid too much attention to it.

"If you were in bad shape, which is, of course, the reason you went there in the first place, they also made an attempt to get the exacerbation under control. The goal was to put out the fire so you could get things back together. I doubt that when I was feeling that bad I would have listened to him anyway. When your body's going crazy on you, you're not interested in someone telling you that if you eat right, you'll feel better."

Suzanne shakes her head.

"I know that. If he hadn't gotten the symptoms under control right there in the beginning, I probably wouldn't have gone any further. I can't say that for sure. But when things started quieting down and I got back to being more normal, I realized I believed in what this guy was doing. (I shouldn't call him that. He's not just a guy; he's a doctor, like you, Peter.) He explained to me that what he had done was to treat my bladder infection and that I probably got the infection because of MS—I didn't know when my bladder was empty, which left a residue of urine for the bacteria to breed in. He explained the connection with endotoxin, a lot of which I didn't understand, but when he got onto the foods, I began to realize that he was offering me a chance. I'm not sure exactly why I took it, except that he had helped me so far. I guess I decided it was worth giving it a try. Nobody else had offered me any help.

"The treatment I received consisted of five elements. Suzanne starts to tick off the five parts with her fingers. *"Control the infection, get the exacerbation under control,*

find out your food allergies, develop a diet, and get into some kind of physical therapy. We also had those consciousness-raising groups, which helped a lot. When you're from a small town there may not be anyone else around with MS. It's nice to talk with someone who knows what's bothering you. All the patients in the hospital while I was there—and I ended up there three times, because I didn't take care of myself well enough—received the same treatment."

Samuels finishes his tea.

"With me it was different; fifteen years ago, they were working on new treatment techniques, but it was kind of every patient for himself. How could it have been any different? Our treatment was based on the conventional knowledge at that time, which amounted to, 'We don't know enough, so let's be careful about what we do.' I do wish they could have done more for me then. I feel like I've missed a lot."

The treatment that Suzanne Baccone received was based on controlling the exacerbation of her disease, treating the mechanism that caused the flare-up—infection—and then prescribing a diet that eliminated her food allergies. These steps reduced the further absorption of endotoxin and/or access of other food allergens into the bowel wall.

With patients such as Suzanne, control of neurological symptoms, if necessary, was accomplished using corticosteroids or ACTH. People who recommend an extremely conservative approach have not favored the use of either. Having the pharmaceutical therapy available to help control MS exacerbations made it possible, however, to clear up the inflammation in the central nervous system and give the dietary modification program a chance to work. It is an attack on two fronts. You achieve immediate results by eliminating the infection or whatever other source of endotoxin may be contributing to the exacerbation. Then you reduce the acute allergic inflammation in the body—especially in the central nervous system—with the help of steroids, if necessary. Finally you maintain this control by limiting the sources of endotoxin. The latter can be achieved, to a large extent, through general control of infections and dietary modification.

Adrenal-cortical-tropic-hormone (ACTH) is a protein our bodies manufacture in the pituitary gland at the base of the brain. It stimulates the adrenal glands to secrete cortisone as well as several other hormones. If ACTH is administered in an intramuscular injection, as a gel preparation, because the entire dose enters the body at once, much of it is destroyed before it has a chance to work. If it is provided intravenously, however, it is possible for the patient to receive almost the full benefit of the dose. The medication is provided in an IV bottle, drop by drop, producing a measured but constant stimulation of the adrenal gland to secrete the cortisone, which in some way apparently calms the inflammatory reaction of MS. Thus the body does not receive a direct injection of additional cortisone, but rather is stimulated to increase production of its own natural hormones. The resulting increased cortisone acts generally to suppress inflammation, including the ongoing inflammation that occurs as a result of the interaction between the white blood cells and the central nervous system tissue. Theoretically, it should be pointed out, however, that the anti-inflammatory effects of cortisone on the central nervous system may in part be secondary to suppression of inflammation in the intestinal wall.

Suzanne looks up from her teacup.

"But Dr. Soll told me that he didn't like to use ACTH because it masked the food allergy reaction. You eat something to which you're allergic, which causes inflammation in your GI tract, and then ACTH suppresses the reaction. This means you can go on eating the foods you shouldn't without realizing that you're hurting yourself."

"That's correct, Suzanne, which is why Dr. Soll will administer ACTH only to control an acute exacerbation. Otherwise, your symptoms might be controlled temporarily, but the primary mechanism for causing the incident would not be affected," Peter Samuels replies.

Samuels gets up and starts pacing around the room.

"It's like people who take medication for high blood pres-

sure. What they usually get is a medication that flushes the extra water out of their body. This means, in effect, that they have less fluid in their system and less pressure, so their blood pressure reading goes down. It's kind of a stopgap measure. What it does is allow them to continue the habits that contributed to developing high blood pressure in the first place. Their medication doesn't do anything to help their disease, but it does control the symptoms.

"So Dr. Soll has been judicious about using ACTH to stimulate our production of natural cortisone. His real interest is in controlling infection and getting people started on an allergen-free regimen. In my discussions with him he indicated that he believes that administration of steroids is for acute problems, and that the real solution is relatively simple: stop the source of endotoxin and you'll reduce the symptoms of MS. You realize, of course, that using steroids like ACTH doesn't help very much if you don't also control the infection. I believe he's correct, but you do get people who continue to smoke, or won't eliminate a favorite food, or refuse to take responsibility for their actions. They think that their life will be awful if they have to modify their habits. I'd describe it as an attitude of 'Well, I want to live life to the fullest while I can, and I'll just take the consequences as they come.' If it were a quick death, I could see it.

"But you know, we abuse our health terribly in this country. Those people like us, who are ill, too often take other people who appear to be healthy as standards for measuring themselves. Very often these people are doing all the wrong things—overeating, not exercising, drinking too much, and exposing themselves to too much stress. Maybe we don't have it so bad after all. Perhaps the way we live is the way everyone should be living. We do it because we have to—because it keeps our disease under control. My thought is that this food allergy business is more important than just us. My guess is that a lot of people have problems they live with every day and never even think might be related to food. But, anyway, if you get on the diet and watch the infections and generally turn out to be a knowledgeable person about your health, you probably won't need any medication. What you're doing if

you do take it when you're in really bad shape is buying yourself the time to get your act together and get better."

Suzanne stares at Peter for a long time before she says anything, then she laughs.

"I'm glad we're talking about these things, Peter, because I've been thinking about this for a while now. I read a lot, not always about MS or even medicine; sometimes religious and inspirational books, sometimes even self-help things. I've read a couple of books about food allergies which have speculated about other problems they might be related to. I believe it. Because I've noticed that, since I've been rotating my diet, some of the other things that were bothering me have disappeared. I used to have what I thought were sinus headaches; I don't have them anymore, unless I get into my chocolate really heavy; and backaches—I never have backaches anymore."

Now she is up, walking toward the window. It has started to snow.

"When I was in the hospital, I took Vivonex to clean out my system, just like all the other patients, and after four days we started to add back food. It took a couple of days to find some foods I could tolerate so I'd have something to live on when I went home. I needed time to get my bearings, which I did. Everyone there went through the same process. You would see people come in who were in really bad shape, in a wheelchair, so depressed and feeling awful. I went in blind once; I couldn't see out of one eye for two weeks. We'd get our history taken and our system cleaned out and start to be human again.

"As soon as we could move they sent us down to physical therapy. The people there knew about the problems of MS patients, and they really worked with us, not just to get us to a certain point but to push us as far as we could go. I know they used to talk to Dr. Soll and tell him when they thought we weren't working hard enough. I hated physical therapy at first, but I understand now why I need it."

Peter gets another cup of tea and joins Suzanne at the window. It's snowing heavily now. He says:

"I never had any physical therapy early in my illness. I wish

I had, because it would have made it much easier for me to get around. I think it's an absolutely essential part of the treatment because, as you get better neurologically—so that your nerves start to function again—it's really good to get working on the muscles and joints. You need to stretch the tightness out. After you've been lying in bed for a while, whether it's because of MS or anything else, you're like jelly. I was in pretty good shape originally because I had been an athlete in college and had worked hard in the service. My muscles got mushy, however, and I think that physical therapy would have helped. Maybe then I could have played football with my son. I have pushed hard, however, by insisting that I do as much as I can for myself. Going places independently, forcing my muscles to work, has given me a great physical as well as psychological boost. I'm not sure that helps the reflexes, though, and that's where physical therapy is a good thing. Of course, if you don't treat the neurological symptoms, the patient can't make much use of the physical therapy."

Suzanne agrees:

"That's where MS patients can become confused. They are told to go out and push themselves. How can they? Their nervous system still won't operate correctly. They tell a muscle to do something and there's no reaction. They don't have the control they need. Once you get your disease into remission and get things quieted down by keeping yourself healthy and watching the irritating foods, then you can get down on the mat and do something physical. I know Janet Myerson really got into that as soon as she came home from Waterloo. That's why she's in such good shape now. She started right away, as soon as she got the diet going. She didn't wait around and say, 'Oh, I've had all these other problems; the last thing I want to do is sweat.' "

Peter turns from the window and walks back across the room to the table.

"I was a basket case when I started on the food allergy plan, so I guess I was lucky. I've seen people in wheelchairs who've done nothing with their disease because they didn't know they could. And then they go on this regimen, and after a few

weeks they can stand up out of their wheelchairs and walk a little bit, holding on to something. Two years later, they might not have gained much further, but they haven't gotten any worse. That's got to feel awfully good. You're slipping downhill, and then the spiral stops. In my case that's what happened. I wasn't in a wheelchair yet, but my balance was off and I couldn't always control my legs. Now I'm OK with that. Of course, one thing that helped—I'm almost ashamed to mention that it took me so long to do it—I stopped smoking."

Suzanne laughs and says, *"That's another thing I also had a problem with. It took me a while, too, Peter, and I've watched a lot of people struggle with quitting."*

Peter continues, *"Dr. Soll thinks I'm still coming back, and that I'll get back even further. But you can't fool around with it. It's taken a lot a work. Suzanne, you are very fortunate; you got the word right in the beginning. I hope you realize that you have a special responsibility to keep it. You should become a personal ambassador to anyone who gets MS. Get to them immediately. Tell them, 'Don't get depressed; don't run around in circles. Just get right down to watching your health. Don't do a bunch of crazy things because you feel sorry for yourself. Go right ahead and get control of this thing.'"*

"You know, Peter, I watched some of the people who were in the hospital with me and some of the people whom I've talked to about my treatment since then. The people who are doing well are the ones who made a decision to conquer their disease. In the hospital we all talked a lot. I heard some people tell Dr. Soll one thing about what they were doing and tell me another. They would cheat and not admit it, but there wasn't much he could do. He couldn't give them any more medication. I'm sure that he was disappointed that they didn't do better. He spent a great deal of time talking to us and listening to our symptoms and how we lived, but he couldn't go home with us.

"If he has a fault as a doctor, it's that he took people too much at their word. He didn't question what they told him. But then again, it's their responsibility, I guess. It was a very

close relationship we all had with Dr. Soll and the staff in the hospital. Either you were smart enough to take advantage of it or you weren't. I know there are reasons people didn't, but it's too bad. Maybe they did better with their own doctor. They didn't have to go to a neurologist after they left the hospital. They could always go right back to a specialist, and he could help them with their infections and monitoring their diet."

The treatment Suzanne and other patients received followed a specific program. Those who came to the clinic soon after they were diagnosed and who were not severely incapacitated were treated by controlling any infections they might have had. Then they were put on a program to identify the allergens in their environment, especially food allergies, which they were taught to avoid. They were also conditioned to evaluate other possible allergens they might be living with unknowingly. In order to clean out their systems so they could test for allergy, they were given the Vivonex for four days. If the individual had severe symptoms, and if he or she was experiencing an acute exacerbation at the time, a ten day course of intravenous ACTH was given. The longer the individual had suffered with MS, the more dramatic the improvement was. Likewise, the sooner the patient was put on a dietary modification program, usually the quicker and more dramatic was the recovery.

Physical therapy is an essential component of this program and was undertaken simultaneously with the other aspects of treatment. Again, those people who didn't delay in obtaining treatment and embraced the physical therapy usually experienced the most gains. The goal was to get them into a program they could maintain when they got home.

Patients were successful to the degree that they took responsibility for themselves and worked with the staff available to them. It was an important part of the program that, during their hospital stay, they could socialize with other multiple sclerosis patients and have access to psychological therapists who helped them address the social and/or emotional problems which can be associated with their disease. Each element of the program was essential. Without the control of infection and the related significant reduction in the release of endotoxin, dietary modification wouldn't have been sufficient to control their MS. If acute exacerbations were not alleviated, both physical strength and willpower were considerably diminished. All of these required the cooperation of the patient, for whom the consciousness-raising groups helped develop the necessary motivation.

Treating a disease as complicated as multiple sclerosis, particularly at this stage of our understanding, is not a single-step process. We do not yet have the luxury of some miracle cure that will control the symptoms and keep the disease in remission. Each component of the treatment program was interrelated with the others, and its effectiveness depended on the patient's attitude. The physician can do only so much, and if the patient is not willing to cooperate, that can never be enough. If the two can work together as a team, however, the possibilities are infinite.

14

MS PATIENTS ARE PEOPLE, TOO

Discussing the new girlfriend of a just divorced associate, a friend said, "Of course she's different from you and me. At twenty-one she still has all her options open." We laughed together over the phone—both of us all of thirty-two—like two conspiring old hags that had let life pass them by.

Most of us start off viewing life as an immense canvas of promise and opportunity. A lot of what we read and see reinforces this concept. The process of growing up, however, is one of defining options, of narrowing our canvas to a manageable size on which we may achieve our hopes and dreams. Maturity comes with realizing that not all the things we dreamed about will come true and that individually we may not be capable of filling all the shoes we've considered for ourselves. This is not a negative process, but rather the product of an enlightened mind which has come to know itself well and is able to effect compatibility between its aspirations and its actual potential.

That life is fluid is an unavoidable conclusion. The secret, as the generation of the sixties reminded us, is knowing how to "go with the flow." Our needs, desires, and priorities necessarily change over the course of a lifetime. What seemed important a few years ago may be fading, perhaps to return again in another guise several years hence. This process has been beautifully described by sociologist William Maslow and has become widely and informally known as Maslow's hierarchy of needs. The system has become so fundamental to sociological thought that it is one of the first theories students encounter and yet still routinely provides the framework for the work of more advanced scholars.

What Maslow developed was a description of the stages we pass through in our efforts to manage our lives. He divides human behavior into seven stages, briefly summarized below:

Ultimate Actualization of one's potential
Self-actualization
Esteem
Love
Belonging
Safety
Basic physiological needs

What Maslow theorized and documented is an extremely accurate scheme for understanding the scope, intensity, and direction of human effort. Each of us starts at the bottom and inches determinedly toward the top. Some of us make it further than others. Each level of effort depends on the successful achievement of those that precede it. This might seem self-evident—that one would have little thought of self-fulfillment if he were homeless and hungry. Indeed, we are, all of us, initially propelled by the needs of food, clothing, and shelter—the ultimate necessities. Satisfied that we will have enough to eat, a place to sleep, and clothes to ensure the opportunity for social interaction, we must then protect what we have acquired. This is a need that will continue to manifest itself as our priorities develop from necessities to luxuries. What we seek to protect, however, is not just the material manifestations of our effort but the feeling of place, security, and continuity symbolized by achievement of this level.

Satisfaction and guarantee of these "basic" needs open the way for expansion of our efforts. Anyone who is a prisoner of unemployment or who is living off the benevolence of others would be blocked at this level. His strategy for providing life's necessities is tentative and temporary at best and will continue to preoccupy him until he develops a permanent and predictable solution.

Home base established and secure, however, we are encouraged to venture into the world, seeking the social interaction necessary to assuage our need for belonging. This compulsion to belong to a group or to be categorized as a group member is related to the desire for increased security, a sense of identity, and it is the initial step toward characterization of self—a process that hopefully we will continue to nurture throughout our lifetime.

By now you should appreciate how each of these levels is self-reinforcing and mutually interdependent. That is, you can't go on to the next step until the previous one has been accomplished. It is not unlike the process by which man developed civilization. In the beginning, given the level of his expertise at the time, primitive man was forced to expend the bulk of his energies on staying alive—feeding himself, securing temporary shelter, and defending his small gains from intruders. He lived a basically antisocial existence, dependent primarily on himself, his personal resources, and those of his immediate family. There was little group cooperation and thus a great deal of independent behavior. As the years passed and he developed his tools and skills, man learned the virtues of interdependence and the rewards of settling down. Eventually people began to develop roles based on their work—farmer, merchant, craftsman, soldier. These roles facilitated the accomplishment of tasks and contributed to the development of both individual and group identity. This in turn produced a corresponding sense of belonging with groups of other people perceived as similar to oneself.

It was inevitable that small settlements would expand until

they coalesced into cities to accommodate the demands of an ever more sophisticated and intertwined social structure. With the cities, many of which started as market towns, came the necessity of defense and the accompanying sense of territorial rights, which expanded far beyond the small nomadic settlements where man originally lived. Only after cities were established and protected and commerce and trade assured did man have enough leisure time and energy to develop the finer things of life—art and culture for example. With that, civilization as we know it began.

Likewise, until you succeed in satisfying your basic needs, you will, of necessity, remain preoccupied with them. There is no way around it; the effort is basic to your survival. Among the "basic" needs we include that of belonging— which we have already mentioned—and love. The need to be loved can occupy a lifetime of effort and, as such, is perhaps one of the most significant and abused sidetracks on which we humans stumble. Unless this need is satisfied to some extent, there seems to be little chance that the individual will become whole enough to pursue the higher levels of human effort necessary for the pursuit of esteem and self-fulfill-ment. If we do not feel that we are valuable and perhaps essential to others, our entire sense of self-worth can be threatened. Incidentally, this does not necessarily mean the love in a one-to-one relationship. We are referring to a much more generalized phenomenon, which includes acceptance of personal significance and the exchange of care and concern with others.

Esteem and fulfillment seem to be rooted in a variety of different areas of effort. Basically, we all want to be well thought of by our primary reference groups—those around us whose opinions we value. For a college student, this may be a social group such as a sorority or fraternity; for a housewife, her circle of friends; for an employee, the hierarchy in the organization for which he/she works or a group of his/her peers. We strive for the acknowledgment that our efforts have paid off and that other individuals recognize them. Esteem, like love, can become a lifelong search. If for some reason it proves to be elusive, it can become preoccupying and distracting, inhibiting other efforts toward self-fulfillment.

It is difficult to say what self-fulfillment is, but it seems to involve successful satisfaction of all of the needs we have discussed thus far, combined with some stretching. For purposes of this discussion, let us consider it an essential factor in pursuing the top of the needs pyramid—the ultimate maximization of our potential as an individual. Let us further describe it as achieving the optimum balance between our dreams and our capabilities.

The urgency of our needs for achievement, esteem, and belonging may block our efforts toward self-fulfillment, as in the case of an executive who sacrifices emotional satisfaction for financial gain or an artist who trades notoriety for integrity. Reaching our ultimate potential involves just that—reaching and stretching far beyond the immediate satiation of our concern for security and safety—if only temporarily. Many, many, many of us never attain it.

In its general manifestations the process we have just described often parallels the chronological life of an individual, although it may be interrupted at any stage, as, for example, in a person who decides on a career change. Motivated by the perceived need for self-fulfillment and secure in his success up to that point, he may find that "starting over" lands him back at level three or four, and he is faced again with assuaging his needs for belonging and recognition. Depending on his planning and the PR campaign he mounts for those around him, he may also find himself jostling with the puzzled stares of family and friends who were comfortable in their adjustment to him as he was. Similar challenges may confront an individual struggling to adjust to the loss of a loved one, a divorce, or an unexpected job change.

Individuals who find themselves diagnosed with MS would know the feeling. Discovering his MS, an individual who has been humming along in his life may feel like the bottom has suddenly dropped out. He may unexpectedly be forced to cope with unwanted feelings of isolation, lack of love, and low esteem.

"I'm not board-certified you know. They think I'm going to die." The remark stings in its intensity. Years of frustration and dissatisfaction linger in these words. But then Peter Samuels' face softens. Light shines. *"But I won't give it up. I'm reading better, and I'll try it again. You have to work with what you have. I'm not bitter. Everyone has their opinion, but I'm not bitter."* Peter climaxes his remarks by slamming his fist down hard on the table.

Although he has conquered his MS, Peter has not yet regrouped to a point that he's satisfied with. His dreams of medicine were nipped in the bud, one of the most cruel effects of MS. He has spent years chipping away at the forces which have compromised his effort. And he has been successful. His wife has stood by him; his children are growing and maturing and are successful in their own lives.

But it has not been easy, and Peter's sense of frustration is associated with the fact that, as he has struggled toward self-fulfillment, he has been forced to be continually preoccupied with the necessities of life. Because of the restrictions posed by their illness, MS patients often must drop back and deal with aspects of living that most of us have probably long passed by and take for granted. The necessities of food, clothing, and shelter may have to be rethought if the individual finds himself unable to walk without assistance, fix his own meals, or even earn his own living. It is a harrowing fall—from a life that is well-ordered and on its way to dealing with needs that one thinks have long ago been taken care of. Depending on his attitude, a person could get stuck in these concerns, becoming more and more incapacitated, necessitating further and more intense preoccupation at the lower levels of human effort.

Fortunately, there are other opportunities, secondary gains, as Samuels calls them. For Peter, one of those gains has been the development of what he calls an informed perspective on his profession. Multiple sclerosis has kept him from throwing himself full force into medicine, as he once envisioned he would. Some years he could hardly work; during others he has had to cut down because of lack of stamina. The benefit of his reduced work load has been extra "think" time, and Peter has in measure used it to ponder his profession. His scrutiny has produced the conclusion that in many ways medicine has come up short for him, as both a physician and a patient. Currently Peter is evaluating his future direction and the nature of his commitment as a doctor. His children are growing up with the result that his degree of financial responsibility will be diminished. His experiences with MS have interested him in a total-person, humanistic approach to illness. His own discoveries about the influence of lifestyle on health and well-being have convinced him that factors such as diet, exercise, and stress can be as important in influencing the health of an individual as treatment with drugs and technology.

"I would like to do something along the lines of what Dr. Soll has done," he says. *"I'm becoming increasingly disenchanted with medicine as I see it. I must say that this may be because I have not experienced the gains I might have professionally if I'd been able to work at peak levels like I once thought I wanted to. Don't mistake me; I'm not advocating that we chuck the whole thing; truly, we need the arsenal of drugs and surgical techniques and diagnostic equipment we've developed. I think what I object to is their dominance in medicine today, their hold over the physician."*

Samuels continues to develop his thoughts.

"It may be that my experiences have produced a new perspective for myself. I think it is really that I see a void. Patients need the friendly voice, the soothing hand of the physician, the sensitivity of his heart and soul, person to person. I'd like to be able to offer patients something like that. And education—the average person just doesn't know enough about his body and how to take care of it."

The point is that, once you get your MS under control, you can and should get on with your life. The problems and challenges brought about by the disease may perhaps provide clues to establishing a direction. Even as you work to install your diet, get yourself back into shape, and plan your new health regimen, you need to give some thought to your goals and aspirations. As many people with MS have done, you may have lowered or drastically reduced your expectations, fearing that you might never again have the opportunity to excel. Somewhere along the way you may have blocked yourself emotionally as protection against disappointment and failure. It gets back to the argument we presented earlier. You are a person who has been stricken with MS; that's it. Where you go after that realization and after you implement your program to control the disease is up to you.

But where do you go? How do you pick up the pieces? First of all, recognize how far you've come—from a person who was looking at life down the narrow pipe of disability to someone who has the capability to hang on for the duration. In early chapters we indicated that MS typically hits people in their twenties and thirties. You were probably well on your way—experimenting and narrowing your options, initiating action and receiving feedback, trying to facilitate that peculiar combination of dreams and capabilities. Go back to that. Where were you when you were interrupted?

Suzanne Baccone was a small-town housewife with two children who were the pride of her life and a voluntary job in the local grade school. Because of her disease, she spent long hours and days away from her family, a thing she would never have thought of doing otherwise. She survived, and so did they. Because of her husband's difficulty in handling her condition, she sought psychiatric help. This was perhaps a turning point, because her therapy helped her discover a stronger sense of her self and put into perspective her own actions and those of others.

She was disqualified from disability payments because she had been so successful with her efforts to control her MS. She then found herself unable to secure any other type of insurance for herself or her family. Unexpectedly and unceremoniously, she was forced into the job market. She says she would have gone to work anyhow, but that she wasn't prepared for the challenge just yet.

Her efforts to secure a job and her encounters with the "system" that denied her insurance have had the effect of radicalizing and sensitizing her to the problems of handicapped workers generally, along with people with chronic disease.

Suzanne explains her frustration.

"If we could just get everyone, not just families and friends but the general public, to have a better understanding of what MS is all about, it would be a lot easier on us. It's probably the same with other diseases. In this country we persist in the impractical belief that everyone is healthy and whole and happy. If you have the least little thing wrong with you, which means you don't fit the image, you're banished to a shell of a life. Handicapped people have needs and desires and goals, too. They should be given a chance. People need the support of their doctors and their families. We need them to truly understand MS and what you can do about it—like me. Then we could go out into the world with the emotional support of a lot of different groups and types of people—employers included. We wouldn't have this feeling of just drifting along. MS people are no different from anyone else; we want to work and be fulfilled. Who wants to sit home amd watch soap operas? Not me."

Suzanne also suffered the financial difficulties that too often confront people with chronic illness. Her problems went beyond her own health needs. No one in Suzanne's family can get major medical insurance because of her MS.

"We've provided health profiles for the whole family and documentation that MS isn't inherited. But they still won't give it to us, no matter what we're willing to pay. I don't want any favors; I just want to be treated fairly. At first the whole business of losing disability was enough to get me out marching. The physician who examined me to determine if I still 'have MS' wasn't even a neurologist. It doesn't leave you with much faith in the system."

Given her own difficulties and her sense of the implications for others, Suzanne could conceivably develop the cause of the handicapped worker as an avocation. It would be an excellent combination of her expanded consciousness as an MS victim and her desire to "make a contribution." A warm, sensitive person who is also very personable and outgoing, there is little doubt that she has felt a great deal of self-satisfaction and fulfillment from her interaction with other MS victims. The ability to commiserate with people and help share their burdens is a skill she might not have developed if it weren't for her MS. Indeed, her capabilities are such that she might want to consider a career in the counseling area.

Suzanne sees her whole life as a contribution to understanding multiple sclerosis. *"I'm thinking of the fact that I have children of my own and they'll have children. I don't want this to happen to anybody else if it doesn't have to, because they may not be as lucky as I was."*

Suzanne's MS has taught her about herself and her relationships with others in a way she could never have imagined possible when she called the information operator years ago on a dark winter morning. The fact that she can implement strategies to control her condition has given her confidence in other areas of her life. Unquestionably, her experiences have strengthened her.

"An average day, are you kidding?" Janet Myerson looks incredulous. *"Well, I get up about 6:45 A.M. and get dressed. Usually Jamie comes running in because he has to go to the bathroom. Then I get him dressed and check to make sure Sarah is ready. She's in first grade and usually manages OK herself, but if I'm running late I'll help her. I give the kids breakfast and stuff something into my mouth if I have time or else I'll grab a piece of fruit or something. Then I leave. We're usually out of the house by 8:00. I drop Sarah off with a neighbor, who watches a couple of the kids until it's time for them to go to school. Then I take Jamie to nursery school and make sure he gets his lunch lined up. Then I go to work.*

"Work is about ten minutes away and four flights up. I work as a therapist with learning-disabled teenage kids. I love it; it's the greatest job I've ever had—those kids. I try to teach them a little English and history and some science and math. Some days I just end up listening to their problems and why they're there. I work part-time—four hours a day. With everything else I have to do, that's enough.

"After work, I pick up my son at the daycare center and go home. Sarah comes home from school in the afternoon; sometimes she goes out, sometimes she plays at home and I

do my exercises. If she goes to a friend's, I'll go out and jog, then I usually make myself something to eat and then get dinner. By that time Nat will be home. I set up my schedule so that I work three days a week. Wednesdays and Fridays are my days. Fridays are swimming days and Wednesdays are for food shopping and the other treats I want to do for myself. Which I do. If I feel like having a manicure, I'll do it."

Cindy Morse smiles shyly. *"What do I do on an average day? I don't have any children, so I guess that probably makes it easier."* She laughs, *"I do have that big dog. I like to experiment. I get up in the morning and do the exercises I learned in the hospital. They're probably not strenuous enough but I do them. Then I have breakfast and do my housework—the usual stuff. If I have time, I'll do some crewel work or my embroidery, some crocheting. Those are my big things. I can't stand on my feet too long, so when I feel like my legs might give out on me, I just sit down and rest.*

"What I've really gotten into is cooking. I like to experiment with food, and having to watch my diet because of the MS has led me into a whole different thing, collecting allergy recipes.

"Who knows why life happens the way it does? You just have to make the best of it. Come to think of it, maybe that's the wrong way to think of it. Maybe you find opportunities where you least think to look. Maybe I should write an allergy cookbook."

Janet, as usual, has the last word.

"Remember how I told you I could always talk? Well, now you know what I said was true. I don't mind talking about MS. I think I'm a living example that you can beat it. Once you've made a commitment, you can and should help yourself as well as you can. I know there are all degrees of MS, but I think that the more determined you are to help yourself and to do what you have to do, the better your chances are. I really do.

"A woman called me the other day and asked me if I would go out again canvassing for MS. I told her I couldn't now because I have MS and I didn't think I'd be strong enough to do it. Actually I think it would be a little awkward—all my neighbors know I have multiple sclerosis; it would seem like collecting money for myself.

"Now, the Cancer Society, that's another story."

EPILOGUE:
WHERE DO WE
GO FROM HERE

MS remains a mystery. But we are inching closer to discovering where the clues are buried. Thus far we have put to good use the implements we possess to carry forth the search, and our preliminary maps have suggested logical routes. Slowly, we are eliminating the detours. Experiences from previous travelers have helped clarify the search. Gradually, we find that our tools need refining, and our maps require more detail. Large dark areas still exist. Our energy, however, remains high. As does our optimism. We are closer than ever before.

Among our tools, our tests for determining food allergies must be rethought and redesigned so we can determine direct correlations between ingestion of specific foods and an individual's symptoms. We must come to a better understanding of food intolerance. Is it actually a classical allergy, or does it result from problems associated with the digestive process? Current diagnostic procedures are inadequate and confusing. Until we have better tests, it will be difficult to do controlled studies, and the whole area will remain in shadow. But it is a fruitful route and warrants further investigation.

The pulse and niacin tests could be used to determine an individual's irritating foods and then patients followed as they are maintained on an allergen-free diet and matched against a control group of patients who continue to eat their allergic foods.

Another clue that should be investigated is our understanding of the nature of food. It would be a crucial step forward to know more about the chemical composition of our raw food and how it breaks down during the digestive process. Are there common chemicals shared by allergic foods? Is an individual who's allergic to corn and bananas actually reacting to the same or similar chemicals? Are there foods that none of us should eat?

And the great mystery of endotoxin. It would be extremely informative if we had a method by which to measure the amount of endotoxin circulating in a person's blood—at various times and in response to specific circumstances. Perhaps this is a challenge for basic science. Does an enzyme regulate the action of endotoxin? Could that enzyme be missing at the site of the MS plaques in the central nervous system?

And the immune system, still the most dense territory of all, perhaps houses the most fundamental mysteries. How much more is there for us to learn about how the white blood cells accomplish their work? How many more functions of white blood cells will we discover as we continue the search? Can we control their reactions and thus allergies? Will their secrets lead to conquering MS?

Will we finally pinpoint a virus as playing a substantive part in the disease? And what will that be? And what of interferon and prostaglandins? Is basic myelin protein the causative antigen? If so, what particular element initiates the immune system's attack?

Of course, there must be the controlled studies. Even with our less than adequate tools, we can accomplish them now. More than any clinical work currently being considered in the area of MS, we need to clarify the relationship among containing infection, the release of endotoxin, and an exacerbation of multiple sclerosis. Why do we see such varied patterns of the illness? Are there different mechanisms at work? Controlled studies could help provide the answers. At the very least, they could generate possible hypotheses for the basic scientists. Above all, let us accomplish something with patients who are prepared to experiment rather than sit and hope and wait.

Patient education is another goal. These patients have demonstrated the value of including themselves, and even their families, in the treatment process. They want and need more information about their illness, and given that information, they are amazingly prepared to take responsibility for their part in getting well. There are no magical solutions to any health problem. Our body is a complex machine, and when it breaks down it requires aid on a number of fronts.

There is a significant difference between medicine and health. What we know of the science of medicine can be applied to an individual when he's ill and in some cases— such as innoculation—to prevent him from illness. Health is another matter; it is an approach to life that considers the strength and the weakness of the human organism in its susceptibility to illness and disease and seeks to implement strategies to prevent both. Multiple sclerosis is a case in point.

It is a fascinating world, this universe of the human body. Let us continue to study it, to heal it, to respect it. Above all, let us continue to search for the clues and take our challenges from whence they come.

FOOTNOTE
REFERENCES

CHAPTER THREE

1. "New Way to Help Multiple Sclerosis Victims Cope," *U.S. News and World Report,* Vol. 86, January 8, 1979, p. 45.
2. Soll, R. W., "The Enigma of Multiple Sclerosis," *Postgraduate Medicine,* Vol. 52, No. 4, Oct., 1972, pp. 113–18.
3. Kurland, Leonard, T., "An Appraisal of Population Studies of Multiple Sclerosis," *Annals of the New York Academy of Sciences,* Vol. 122, March 31, 1965, pp. 520–41; Fischman, Harvey R., "Multiple Sclerosis: A New Perspective on Epidemiologic Patterns," *Neurology,* Vol. 32, August, 1982, pp. 864–70.
4. Haspel, M. V., Lampert, P. W., and Oldstone, M. B. A., *Proceedings of the National Academy of Science,* USA, Vol. 75, 1978, pp. 4033–36.
5. Soll, R. "Delayed Hypersensitivity—A Possible Mechanism in Me Etiology of MS," *Epidemiology of MS,* Alter, M. and Kurtzke, J.F., Springfield, IL, Charles C. Thomas, 1968.
6. Schultz, D., "MS: Two New Clues," *Science Digest,* Vol. 86, August, 1979, p. 83.

7. Wang, S., "The Mystery of MS: Who Gets It, Who Doesn't," *New York Magazine*, Vol. 13, March 26, 1979, p. 76.

CHAPTER FOUR

1. Soll, R. W., "Etiology and Progression of MS," *Minnesota Medicine*, Vol. 61, December, 1978, pp. 711–19.
2. A recent study confirms this observation about infection and MS. The study consisted of 251 multiple sclerosis patients. On the basis of a 19-page questionnaire, a complete patient history, and evaluation of present status, each individual was classified as Type I or Type II. Type I consisted of those subjects who had suffered very few recent infections. Type II were those people who had had two or more infectious problems per year throughout their childhood and as adults. Type II patients suffered more symptoms of multiple sclerosis in all spheres than their Type I counterparts. The number of attacks in the first five years was also higher for the former group. Additionally, although the age of onset was the same for both groups, the mean age in Type II was 36 years, while in Type I group it was 46. The authors conclude that MS patients with a history of infections may experience a more rapid and severe development of their disease. See Lamoueux, G., et al, "Effects of Past Infectious Events on Disease Evolution in Multiple Sclerosis," *Journal of Neurology*,

Vol. 230, 1983, pp. 81–90.

CHAPTER FIVE

1. Buisseret, Paul B., "Allergy," *Scientific American*, Vol. 24, No. 2, August, 1982, pp. 86–95. This article provides an excellent introduction to the underlying mechanisms of allergy in understandable layman's terms, as well as discussing clinical effects.

2. Forman, Robert, *How to Control Your Allergies*, Larchmont Books, New York, 1979, pp. 12–35.
3. Coca, Arthur F., *The Pulse Test: Easy Allergy Detection*, Arco Publishing, New York, 1956. Coca's book, written for the lay public, provides a brief overview of the food allergy problem as an introduction to using the pulse test to detect allergies. Coca's more scientific work, *Familiar, Nonreaginic Food-Allergy*, 3rd ed., Charles C. Thomas, Springfield, IL, 1956, provides a more comprehensive discussion of the problem. Forman, in *How to Control Your Allergies*, devotes considerable space to discussing the nature and prevalence of food allergies. For those with a scientific background, *Clinics in Immunology and Allergy*, Vol. 2, Number 1, Jonathan Brostoff and Stephen Challacome, eds., W. B. Sanders Co., Ltd., London, February, 1982, provides a comprehensive discussion of the problem—from the basic mechanism of the reaction, to specific manifestations of food allergies, to reports on treatment.
4. Forman, p. 161.
5. Ibid., p. 158.
6. Feingold, Ben F., *Why Your Child Is Hyperactive*, Random House, New York, 1975. Feingold did the definitive work on hyperactivity in children and this book provides a comprehensive treatment of his views on the subject. See also Forman, pp. 119–51, and Alexander Schauss, *Diet, Crime and Delinquency*, rev. ed., Parker House, Berkeley, 1981, pp. 75–89.
7. Ibid.
8. Ibid.
9. Ibid; also, for a broader discussion of this subject, see Philpott, William H. and Kalita, Dwight, K., *Brain Allergies: The Psycho-Nutrient Connection*, Keats Publishing, Inc., New Canaan, Conn., 1980.
10. Generally noted as fundamental to discussions in: Buisseret, 1982, Brostoff and Challacombe, 1982, Philpott and Kalita, 1980, and Schauss, 1981.
11. Egger, J., et. al., "Is Migraine Food Allergy? A Double-Blind Controlled Trial of Oligoantigenic Diet Treat-

ment," *The Lancet,* Vol. 11, pp. 865–68, 1983; also: Merretl J., et. al., "Food Related Antibodies in Headache Patients," *Journal of Neurology, Neurosurgery, and Psychiatry,* Vol. 46, pp. 738–42, 1983.

12. Monro, J., "Food Allergy and Migraine," Brostoff and Challacombe, pp. 137–46.

13. Forman, p. 194.

14. Mandell, Marshall, "Foreword," Forman, pp. 5–11.

CHAPTER SIX

1. Waksman, Byron, "Current Trends in Multiple Sclerosis Research," *Immunology Today,* May 1981, p. 88.

2. Ibid.; also for a more comprehensive discussion of this subject, see:
   Paterson, Philip Y., "Experimental Allergic Encephalomyelitis and Autoimmune Disease," *Advances in Immunology,* Vol. 5, Academic Press, Inc., New York, 1966, pp. 131–208.
   Weigle, William, O., "Autoimmunity: Thyroiditis and Encephalomyelitis," *Advances in Immunology,* Vol. 30, No. 159, Academic Press, New York, 1980, 159–273.

3. Cremer, Natalie, E., et. al., "Comprehensive Viral Immunology of Multiple Sclerosis," *Archives of Neurology,* Vol. 37, October, 1980, pp. 610–15.

4. Ibid.

5. Grundke-Iqbal, I., et. al., "EAE: Characterization of Serum Factors Causing Demyelination and Swelling of Myelin," *Journal of the Neurological Sciences,* Vol. 50, 1981, pp. 63–79.

6. Bornstein, M. B. and Appel, S. H., "The Application of Tissue Culture to the Study of Experimental 'Allergic' Encephalomyelitis. Patterns of Demyelination," *Journal of Neuropathology and Experimental Neurology,* Vol. 20, 1961, pp. 141–57.

7. Johnson, Kenneth, P., "Cerebrospinal Fluid and Blood Assays of Diagnostic Usefulness in Multiple Sclerosis," *Neurology,* Vol. 30, 1980, pp. 106–9.

8. Pankaj, D. Mehta, Miller, Judith, A., Tourtellotte, Wal-

lace W., "Oligoclonal IgG Bands in Plaques from Multiple Sclerosis Brains," *Neurology*, Vol. 32, 1982, pp. 372–76.

9. Neighbour, P. Andrew, and Bloom, Barry R., "The Interferon-Natural Killer Cell System in Multiple Sclerosis," *Clinics in Immunology and Allergy*, Vol. 2, Number 2, W. B. Saunders, Ltd., London, June, 1982, p. 281.
10. Ibid., p. 284.
11. Ibid., p. 285–86.
12. Ibid., p. 286–87.
13. Droller, M. J., Schneider, M. U., and Perlmann, P., "A Possible Role of Prostaglandins in the Inhibition of Natural and Antibody-dependent Cell-mediated Cytotoxicity Against Tumor Cells," *Cellular Immunology*, Vol. 39, 1978, 165–77.
14. Bloom, B. R., *Nature*, Vol. 287, 1980, 275–76.
15. Dore-Duffy, P. and Zurier, R. B., "Lymphocyte Adherence in Multiple Sclerosis. Role of Monocytes and Increased Sensitivity of MS Lymphocytes to Prostaglandin E.," *Clinical Immunology and Immunopathology*, Vol. 19, 1981, pp. 303–13.
16. Buisseret, p. 93.
17. Weiner, Howard L. and Hauser, Stephen, L., "Cellular Immunological Studies with Monoclonal Antibodies in Neurological Diseases," *Clinics in Immunology and Allergy*, Vol. 2, No. 2, pp. 457–67.
18. Dahlquist, N. R., et al, "D-Lactic Acidosis and Encephalopathy after Jejunoileostomy: Response to Overfeeding and Fasting in Humans," *Mayo Clinic Proceedings*, Vol. 59, pp. 141–45, 1984.
19. Cross, S. A., and Callaway, C. W., "Editorial: D-Lactic Acidosis and Selected Cerebellar Ataxias," *Mayo Clinic Proceedings*, Vol. 59, pp. 202–5, 1984.

CHAPTER SEVEN

1. Coca, *The Pulse Test: Easy Allergy Detection*, pp. 33–50.
2. Ibid, p. 49.
3. Ibid, p. 21.

CHAPTER NINE

1. Watson, David L. and Tharp, Roland G., *Self-Directed Behavior,* Brooks/Cole Publishing, Monterey, 1981. The rationale, as well as the theory and methods of record-keeping, are discussed throughout this book and copious examples are presented.
2. Brightwell, Dennis, R. and Clancy, John, "Self-Training of New Eating Behavior for Weight Reduction," *Diseases of the Nervous System,* 1976, Vol. 37 p. 85; Harris, Mary B., "Self-Directed Program for Weight Control: A Pilot Study," *Journal of Abnormal Psychology,* 1969, Vol. 74, No. 2, pp. 263–70; Jeffrey, Belfour D., "A Comparison of the Effects of External Control and Self-Control on the Modification and Maintenance of Weight," *Journal of Abnormal Psychology,* 1974, Vol. 83, No. 4 pp. 404–10; see also the bibliography in Watson and Tharp.
3. Hirschberg, Leslie D., "Understanding Adherence to Health Behavior Changes: A Review of the Literature," Annenberg School of Communications, University of Southern California, unpublished paper. Hirschberg's bibliography provides a thorough overview of the work in the field of cognitive behavioral modification and self-directed and self-managed change.
4. Watson and Tharp's program for self-directed and self-managed behavior change is described in terms of a system of A-B-Cs—antecedents, behavior, and consequences. Their work is based on current thought in this area and appears to reflect established behavioral strategies.
5. Ibid., pp. 10–18.
6. Ibid., pp. 193–97.
7. Marlot, G., Alan, and Parks, George A., "Self-management of Addictive Disorders" in *Self-management and Behavior Change,* Karoly, P. and Kanfer, F., eds, Pergammon Press, N.Y., 1982, pp. 480–81.
8. Watson and Tharp, pp. 252–56.
9. Watson and Tharp, pp. 176–85.
10. Watson and Tharp, pp. 25–57.
11. Watson and Tharp, pp. 225–49.

CHAPTER ELEVEN

1. Marlot and Parks, pp. 461–64.
2. Marlot and Parks, p. 465; Watson and Tharp, pp. 6–7.
3. Watson and Tharp, pp. 108–9.
4. Ibid., p. 110.
5. Ibid., p. 84.
6. Ibid., p. 251.
7. Ibid., p. 163.
8. Ibid., pp. 127–28, 185–88, 250.

Specific reference is made to the particularly succinct manner in which Watson and Tharp have expressed the necessity of various types of social support. The value of cooperation from one's family, friends, co-workers and other significant others is generally considered essential in programs of self-directed, self-managed change.

CHAPTER TWELVE

1. Although the principle of a balanced lifestyle is not specific to the theory of self-directed and self-managed change, the two primary sources consulted in this area—Watson and Tharp and Marlot and Parks—refer to the necessity of balance, especially in alleviating the types of avoidance behavior typified by over-eating, drug abuse, and alcoholism.

APPENDIX I:
LISTING OF ALLERGY COOK BOOKS

The following books offer additional information about living with food allergies. Although we speculated that health food stores would be a prime source of such information, we discovered the bulk of these books in the local public library.

Coping with Food Allergy, Claude A. Frazier, M.D., Quadrangle/New York Times Book Co., New York, 1974, hardcover, 334 pages.

Of all the books surveyed, this volume presents the most balanced, sensible, informed treatment of the subject. Written in straightforward prose by a physician who is an allergist, it provides an excellent overview of food allergies, including an introduction to the most common allergens, sample menus and recipes. The appendices contain a wide variety of useful information, including a summary of the foods containing the common allergens, the names and addresses of manufacturers of special foods for allergy diets, and additional sources of recipes.

The recipes contained in the main body of the book are organized as to type of food—salads and salad dressings, main dishes, etc.—with each recipe noted as to which antigen it avoids. Dr. Frazier has authored or edited almost twenty books, including two others on the subject of allergies, and his expertise shows. He combines a sense of seriousness with an attitude of hope. An excellent general resource.

The Egg-Free, Milk-Free, Wheat-Free Cookbook, Becky Hamrick and S. L. Wiesenfeld, M.D., Harper and Row, New York, 1981, hardcover, 274 pages.

In his foreword, Dr. Wiesenfeld explains that Mrs. Hamrick developed the recipes contained in the book as a result of discovering that her child was allergic to eggs and milk. The result is an easy-to-read book, laid out like a classical cookbook. It is divided into conventional cookbook sections such as breakfast ideas, appetizers, soups, salads, dressings, sauces, main dishes, etc., and the recipes are well-spaced on the pages so it would be easy to keep this volume in your kitchen and use it as you would an ordinary cookbook. Each recipe is marked by an easy-to-read symbol indicating whether it's egg-, milk- or wheat-free. She does not cover any other types of allergies, however. Nicely illustrated with drawings which add to the pleasantness of the overall presentation.

Recipes for Allergies, Billie Little, Bantam, 1983, paper, 266 pages.

Little developed this book after a lifetime of dealing with her mother's allergies, which included hay fever and numerous food allergies. The book is divided into sections according to the primary allergic foods—eggs, corn, milk, and wheat. There is a short section at the end on other foods such as chocolate. The recipes in each section are grouped according to the number of the primary allergens to which one might be allergic. Thus, the first recipes in the corn section assume an allergy to corn only. Next come recipes for people who are allergic to corn and eggs, then corn and milk, then corn and wheat, then corn, eggs, and milk and so forth. Obviously the author is extremely familiar with her subject. At the back of the book is an excellent section on special food suppliers, along with sources for other recipes and further reading. The entire book is written in a no-nonsense tone and is easy to read.

Do-It-Yourself Allergy Analysis Handbook, Kate Ludeman, Ph.D. and Louise Henderson, Keats Publishing, Inc., New Canaan, Conn., paperback, 154 pages.

This is an interesting book in that it not only presents food recipes for the major food allergies, it contains a sizeable section on making your own natural cosmetics and substitutes for common household cleaners. Regarding food allergies specifically, however, it is not as comprehensive as the other books.

Dr. Mandell's Allergy-Free Cookbook, Fran Gare Mandell, M.S., Pocket Books, New York, 1981, paperback, 252 pages.

The author is the wife of food allergy pioneer Marshall Mandell and also the co-author of *Dr. Atkins' Diet Revolution and Dr. Atkins' Diet Cookbook.* She has a master's degree in biology and clinical nutrition. Her book covers a lot of territory, although not necessarily in detail. She explains the rotary diversified diet, provides examples and recipes. She also presents rotary diets which are corn- and wheat-free; soy-,cane-, and egg-free; and yeast- and milk-free, which should be helpful to people with fixed allergies. Also included are suggestions for lunches, for eating in restaurants, for cocktail parties, and for when on vacation. Altogether, a good, overall guide although some people might be uncomfortable with its upbeat style.

The Allergy Cookbook and Food Buying Guide, Pamela P. Nonken and S. Roger Hirsch, M.D., Warner Books, New York, 1982, paperback, 302 pages.

The design of this book is a little busy and its recipes sometimes difficult to read because of the type and because they often spread over two pages. One interesting addition, however, is a list of commercial products which are free of the major allergens, including corn, eggs, milk, soy, wheat, and yeast, which are the primary allergies treated in the book. Mrs. Nonken started on this project because her daughter is allergic to yeast. Her co-author is an allergist who felt her work should be made available to others. Although the book helps steer the reader toward brand name products that are acceptable and away from those that aren't, it doesn't contain information on alternative sources of food substitutes. You would want to keep these limitations in mind if you are considering buying only one of these books as a reference.

The Allergic Gourmet, June Roth, M.S., Contemporary Books, Chicago, 1983, hardcover, 294 pages.

Roth has an MS in clinical nutrition and has written a number of special diet cookbooks. She explains the rotary diversified diet plan and presents recipes for dairy-free, egg-free and gluten-free diets, as well as a section on multiple allergies. It is a well designed book, breezy yet informative. She also includes a section on menu planning that discusses food group requirements and vitamins. Some illustrations.

Creative Cooking without Wheat, Milk, and Eggs, Ruth R. Shattuck, A.S. Barnes and Company, Cranbury, NJ, 1974, hardcover, 188 pages.

Mrs. Shattuck's book is based on the recipes she developed for her husband, who suffered from a number of food allergies. She is a home economist and has worked in a number of dietary positions in hospitals and dining halls. Her recipes are divided into three parts—breads and deserts, fish and meats, and vegetables and soups. The book is focused on wheat, gluten, milk, and egg allergies. Although the recipes look interesting, they are somewhat difficult to follow if you are used to conventional cookbooks, because instead of listing all the ingredients, followed by directions, she tends to incorporate the two in a procedural format.

APPENDIX II:
FORMS FOR ALLERGY TESTING

On the following pages, you will find blank forms for you to use in doing your own food allergy testing. You may want to cut these pages out and hang them on the refrigerator with the instructions from Chapter 10. As you do your testing, you will need much patience and determination, so keep in mind that the ultimate goal you seek to achieve is the ability to be able to do something about your MS—you *can* do it.

FORM 1—Pulse & Niacin Tests (Regular Diet)

FOODS EATEN Day One	PULSE Pre-Rising	NIACIN REACTION
BREAKFAST		
_____	Premeal _____	
_____	30 min. _____	
_____	60 min. _____	
_____	90 min. _____	
_____	_____	
LUNCH		
_____	Premeal _____	
_____	30 min. _____	
_____	60 min. _____	
_____	90 min. _____	
_____	_____	
DINNER		
_____	Premeal _____	
_____	30 min. _____	
_____	60 min. _____	
_____	90 min. _____	
_____	_____	

FORM 1—Pulse & Niacin Tests (continued)

FOODS EATEN	PULSE	NIACIN
Day Two	Pre-Rising_____	REACTION

BREAKFAST

_____ Premeal_____

_____ 30 min. _____

_____ 60 min. _____

_____ 90 min. _____

_____   _____

LUNCH

_____ Premeal_____

_____ 30 min. _____

_____ 60 min. _____

_____ 90 min. _____

_____   _____

DINNER

_____ Premeal_____

_____ 30 min. _____

_____ 60 min. _____

_____ 90 min. _____

_____   _____

FORM 1—Pulse & Niacin Tests (continued)

FOODS EATEN	PULSE	NIACIN
Day Three	Pre-Rising_____	**REACTION**

BREAKFAST

_____ Premeal _____

_____ 30 min. _____

_____ 60 min. _____

_____ 90 min. _____

_____   _____

LUNCH

_____ Premeal _____

_____ 30 min. _____

_____ 60 min. _____

_____ 90 min. _____

_____   _____

DINNER

_____ Premeal _____

_____ 30 min. _____

_____ 60 min. _____

_____ 90 min. _____

_____   _____

FORM 2—Mini-Meal Tests
(PRE-RISING PULSE——)

FOOD	PULSE				NIACIN
	Premeal	*30*	*60*	*90*	REACTION

FORM 2—Mini-Meal Tests (continued)

(PRE-RISING PULSE_____)

FOOD	PULSE				NIACIN
	Premeal	*30*	*60*	*90*	REACTION

FO RM 3—New Diet

DAY ONE

Breakfast

_____   _____
_____   _____
_____   _____
                           _____

Lunch

_____   _____
_____   _____
_____   _____
_____   _____

Dinner

_____   _____
_____   _____
_____   _____
_____   _____

DAY TWO

Breakfast

_____   _____
_____   _____
_____   _____
_____   _____

Lunch

_____   _____
_____   _____
_____   _____
_____   _____

Dinner

_____   _____
_____   _____
_____   _____
_____   _____

FORM 3—New Diet (continued)

DAY THREE

Breakfast

_____   _____

_____   _____

_____   _____

Lunch

_____   _____

_____   _____

_____   _____

Dinner

_____   _____

_____   _____

_____   _____

_____   _____

DAY FOUR

Breakfast

_____   _____

_____   _____

_____   _____

Lunch

_____   _____

_____   _____

_____   _____

Dinner

_____   _____

_____   _____

_____   _____

FORM 3—New Diet (continued)

DAY FIVE

Breakfast

_____
_____
_____
_____

Lunch

_____
_____
_____
_____

Dinner

_____
_____
_____
_____

DAY SIX

Breakfast

_____
_____
_____
_____

Lunch

_____
_____
_____
_____

Dinner

_____
_____
_____
_____

FORM 3—New Diet (continued)

DAY SEVEN

Breakfast

_____

_____

_____

_____

Lunch

_____

_____

_____

_____

Dinner

_____

_____

_____

_____

INDEX

Abstinence, from allergic foods, 90, 94, 103–4, 123, 130
Accommodation stage of food allergy, 74
Accomplice in self-managed change programs, 121, 134–35, 177–78
Adrenal-cortical-tropic-hormone (ACTH), 4, 8–9, 59, 196, 198, 202
mode of administration, 197
Addiction to allergic foods, 7, 33, 72–74, 94, 101, 129–30, 138, 143
Allergens, 11, 65, 73, 103–4, 144, 196, 198, 202
Allergy. See also Delayed hypersensitivity; Immediate hypersensitivity
classical, 51, 55, 62–63, 71
mechanism of, 67
outgrowing, 74
skin, 62
symptoms of: respiratory, 62
treatment, 63
Allergy cookbooks, 121, 162
American eating habits, 110, 112–13
Antibiotics, 56, 195

Antibodies, 46–48, 82. See also Humoral immunity; Reagins
antigen specific, 81
function of, 42–43
in food allergy testing, 92
monoclonal, 86
Antigenic substance. See Antigens
Antigens, 42–43, 49, 58, 60, 63, 80, 83–85, 101
Antilymphoblastic globulin (ALG), 3–5
Assistance in movement, 20, 29, 186–89, 201, 209
Asthma, 68
Autoimmune Theory of MS, 41–42, 46–49, 78–79, 87
Autoimmunity. See Immune system malfunction
Axon of cell, 45

Bacterial infection, 4–6, 10–12, 39, 43, 56–58, 189, 195–96, 198, 202–3, 216
Basic myelin protein (BP), 79, 216
Behaviorism, 125–26
Blood-barrier system, 54–55, 80
Blood factors, 81
Brain and spinal cord. See Central Nervous System